Aging and Mental Retardation

Monographs of the American Association on Mental Retardation, 9

Michael J. Begab, Series Editor

Aging and Mental Retardation

Extending the Continuum

by

Marsha Mailick Seltzer
School of Social Work
Boston University
and the
Eunice Kennedy Shriver Center

Marty Wyngaarden Krauss
The Heller School
Brandeis University
and the
Eunice Kennedy Shriver Center

Published by
American Association on Mental Retardation
1719 Kalorama Road, NW
Washington, DC 20009

No. 9, Monographs of the American Association on Mental Retardation (ISSN 0895-8009)

Library of Congress Cataloging-in-Publication Data

Seltzer, Marsha Mailick.
    Aging and mental retardation: extending the continuum / Marsha Malick Seltzer and Marty Wyngaarden Krauss.
    p. cm.— (Monographs of the American Association on Mental Retardation. ISSN 0895-8009; 9)
    Bibliography: p. Includes index.
    ISBN 0-940898-18-7 (pbk.): $20.00
    1. Mentally handicapped aged—Services for—United States. I. Krauss. Marty Wyngaarden. II. Title. III. Series: Monographs of the American Association on Mental Retardation; no. 9.
    [DNLM: 1. Health Services for the Aged—United States. 2. Mental Retardation—in old age. W1 M0569QMC no. 9 / WM 300 S468a]
HV3006.A4S45 1987
362.3'0880565—dc19
DNLM/DLC
for Library of Congress   87-27406

Printed in the United States of America

 3

Table
of
Contents

Foreword

In many ways, the aging of America's population of older persons with mental retardation has forced us to "come of age" in terms of how we view the lifespan of this population. This text represents an effort to formulate the types and character of services and programs currently available to older mentally retarded persons as they make the transition from work activities and involvements to those more typical of our nation's senior citizens. The field is young enough not to have institutionalized the available options. Planners, program developers, and administrators still have a wide range of alternatives that they can explore and use to provide effectively and creatively for the needs of their older clientele.

It is clear from this text that the diversity and richness of the options used augers well for the quality of life for aging persons with mental retardation as they seek to re-orient themselves to retirement activities. At the same time, Drs. Seltzer and Krauss present us with the realities and constraints of services both available and unavailable to older citizens who have had to contend with lifelong disabilities. *Aging and Mental Retardation: Extending the Continuum* helps to focus our thinking on how we can avoid some of the pitfalls of the aging network and still draw from the richness of its experiences.

One's later years can be a time when different facets of life can be explored and experienced, when work isn't by necessity the dominant theme in life. The text that Drs. Seltzer and Krauss have prepared is a call to workers in the field of mental retardation to rethink their notions of *clinical appropriateness* regarding how time can best be spent by older and aging individuals with mental retardation. Indeed, the very fact that a person has carried the diagnostic label *mentally retarded* through his or her life becomes less important than the attainment of status as an "older American." The future will see our nation responding to the needs of its older citizens, less by what they bring into old age than by their potential. The same will hold true for the large population of older persons currently in mental retardation services: their disability will become less of a discriminant.

The population demographics are telling. Over the next 30 years, the population of older mentally retarded persons will grow, and dramatically at that. What Drs. Seltzer and Krauss have done in conducting their national survey and in producing this text will enable all of us to be better prepared for the future. What we learn from their work will help this nation to extend the continuum in the most age-appropriate ways.

Matthew P. Janicki

Preface

This monograph examines one segment of the evolving system of services for persons with mental retardation: specialized residential and day programs for elderly mentally retarded persons. The continuum of services has now been extended to cover the full life cycle. With this accomplishment the field of mental retardation, which is affected by the same demographic trends that are characteristic of society at large, has "come of age."

Our interest in studying programs for elderly mentally retarded persons developed directly from our earlier research. About 10 years ago each of us coauthored books about programs for mentally retarded persons. *Coming Back* (Gollay, Freedman, Wyngaarden, & Kurtz, 1978) documented the early progress of the deinstitutionalization movement. *As Close As Possible* (Baker, Seltzer, & Seltzer, 1977) described the emerging community residences service models.

Much has changed during the ensuing 10 years. Whereas 10 years ago few community residences served special populations, the system of community residences has now evolved to the point that it can respond to increasingly specialized subgroups, of which the elderly comprise only one. At the same time, the average age of the residents who have remained in public institutions has increased substantially. Consequently, new services have been developed to meet the needs of the elderly mentally retarded residents in institutional settings as well as in the community.

The National Survey of Programs Serving Elderly Mentally Retarded Persons was conducted in 1984 and 1985 in order to describe the range of programmatic options for this client group. Our intent was to be inclusive rather than exclusive in the scope of the surveyed programs. We made three decisions that broadened the range of the programs we studied. First, we decided to include institutionally based programs in addition to community-based programs because a large proportion of elderly mentally retarded service recipients are residents of public institutions. Second, we decided to include day programs in addition to residential programs because the development of retirement options for elderly mentally retarded persons has emerged as an important and controversial issue for our field. Third, we decided to include programs that served some

ix

younger mentally retarded adults in addition to programs that served elders with mental retardation exclusively because there is no consensus among professionals as to what chronological age should be used to define *elderly* for this population.

At the same time that we increased the heterogeneity of our sample of programs through these three decisions, we chose to limit our study to programs for mentally retarded elders. While mental retardation is only one of many developmental disabilities, we were concerned that the inclusion of programs for nonretarded developmentally disabled elders could introduce a confounding heterogeneity into the sample. Thus, in light of the preliminary stage of our knowledge base about services for elderly mentally retarded persons, we limited our study to programs for this one client group.

Aging and Mental Retardation, Extending the Continuum, then, presents a nationwide perspective on a heterogeneous group of specialized programs for elderly mentally retarded persons. We drew on the results of the quantitative analysis of survey data, direct quotes from respondents, and case examples to highlight various program options for this client group. It has been our goal since the inception of the National Survey to provide planners, service providers, family members, and researchers with baseline data about currently available services so that they can knowledgeably advocate and plan for this latest extension of the continuum.

M.M.S. and M.W.K.

Acknowledgments

The project was lodged in three organizations, reflecting the professional affiliations of the authors. Edwin Kolodny, M.D., Director of the Eunice Kennedy Shriver Center (which assumed administrative responsibility for the project), Hubie Jones, M.S.W., Dean of the Boston University School of Social Work, and Stuart Altman, Ph.D., Dean of the Heller School at Brandeis University, were all steadfast in their enthusiasm for the project and in their understanding of its impacts on our time. It is a privilege to publicly acknowledge the pride we take in being associated with such supportive academic and research institutions.

Gunnar Dybwad, Professor Emeritus at the Heller School, gave his thoughtful encouragement to the project at critical junctures in its development. Mr. and Mrs. Nathan Starr of Toronto, Canada, were generous in their financial backing of the project and in their faith that what we learn in the United States has relevance for other countries. Michael Begab, Ph.D., Editor of the Monograph Series of the American Association on Mental Retardation, was immensely helpful in his critical reviews of drafts of the manuscript and was tolerant of its many delays. We welcome this opportunity to express our gratitude to each of these mentors and supporters.

We relied heavily on the expertise, creativity, and perseverance of our two project managers. Ms. Anne Howard, Project Manager for Field Operations, demonstrated a commitment to excellence and an ability to organize the hundreds of interviews that she supervised. Mr. Leon Litchfield, Project Manager for Data Management and Analysis, mastered the intricacies of our unwieldy dataset. His tolerance of our request for "just one more run, Leon" were indispensable. Both project managers supervised a fleet of graduate students and turned what could easily have been just jobs into educational, intellectually provocative experiences for these students. We are very much in the debt of both project managers for the standards of professionalism that they maintained.

The project attracted a large number of graduate students and other staff from both the Heller School at Brandeis University and the School of Social Work at Boston University. They deserve special credit for their competence in conducting the telephone interviews and processing the data. From the Heller School, we thank Mary Ann Allard, Phyllis Bailey,

xi

Debra Hart, Kenneth Levy, Kristen Magis, Martha McGaughey, Diane Post, and Patty Wilde for their invaluable contributions to the project. From Boston University's School of Social Work, we thank Karen Boebinger, Rhonda Bourne, Madelyn Bronitsky, Charlotte Dickson, Ann Kent, Wayne Kessler, NancyJo Khantzian Modlish, Reva Klepell, Marsha Langer, Chirag Patel, and Sandy Anderson Storer for their careful and diligent work.

Our secretarial staff, Deborah Forbes, Gladys Rivera, and Amy Sheperdson, consistently demonstrated their professional investment in the quality of our printed work by their gracious tolerance of innumerable revisions and, at times, unthinkable deadlines. Marjorie Erickson and Andrea Wingo thoroughly and carefully edited this monograph and substantially improved its readability. We deeply appreciate their collaboration and eye for detail.

The project's success depended heavily on the willingness of people "in the field"—from Commissioners of Aging, Mental Health, and Mental Retardation agencies in the 50 states, to executive directors of large agencies, to operators of individual programs—to answer our questions and offer suggestions to ensure that we discovered as many programs that met our criteria as possible. We are grateful for their time, help, and enthusiasm for the project.

The project received generous support from a wide range of professional organizations and other research institutions. The American Association on Mental Deficiency, the Association for Retarded Citizens-U.S., the Center for Residential and Community Services at the University of Minnesota, the National Association of Private Residential Facilities for the Mentally Retarded, and the National Association of Superintendents of Public Residential Facilities for the Mentally Retarded provided critical assistance to the conduct of this project.

We are also grateful to the multiple funding sources that were tapped (and sometimes, retapped) to complete the project. These include: BRSG RR07044 awarded by the Biomedical Research Support Grant Program, Division of Research Resources, National Institutes of Health (administered by Brandeis University); a supplemental award to grant 03DD 0146/14 from the Administration on Developmental Disabilities to the Eunice Kennedy Shriver Center; a generous grant from the Starr Center for Mental Retardation at the Heller School of Brandeis University; and a grant from the Boston University Intramural Research Program.

Finally, we acknowledge the important role of our families. Our husbands, Gary Seltzer and Richard Krauss, and our children Beth and Rebecca Seltzer and Jake, Rebecca, and David Krauss provided the greatest support of all.

Context for the National Survey of Programs Serving Elderly Mentally Retarded Persons

Chapter 1
Introduction

This monograph presents the results of the National Survey of Programs Serving Elderly Mentally Retarded Persons. The purpose of the survey was to gather information regarding the types, characteristics, and experiences of a wide variety of programs in which older mentally retarded persons live, work, and spend their leisure time. The National Survey focused on community and institutionally based programs serving mentally retarded persons age 55 and over.

Concerns over the needs of mentally retarded persons as they age and about the capacities of existing service systems to meet these needs have been expressed for many years (Butler, 1976; Dybwad, 1962; Hamilton & Segal, 1975; O'Connor, Justice, & Warren, 1970; Sweeney & Wilson, 1979). However, guidelines for the creation or restructuring of programs to meet the varied needs of older and elderly mentally retarded persons have only recently appeared in the literature (Anderson, 1984; Congdon, 1983; Johnson & Olsen, 1982; Mather, 1981). Given the relative infancy of programs serving this target group, it is not surprising that the literature contains little in the way of systematic description or assessment of contemporary programmatic practices of either residential or day services for older mentally retarded persons. In response to this gap in our knowledge base, this monograph presents a national perspective on a diverse and innovative set of programs that, either by design or by evolution, are providing care to a substantial number of mentally retarded persons age 55 and over.

CONTEXT FOR
THE NATIONAL SURVEY

Why is the study of programs for elderly mentally retarded persons important at the present time? One salient factor is our society's recognition of the changing demographic trends affecting all segments of the U.S. population. It is widely recognized that:

- the proportion of our population who are elderly has risen rapidly and will continue to do so;
- the average lifespan is considerably longer than in the past;

- longer life brings with it an increased vulnerability to chronic illness and disability; and,
- there are proportionately fewer younger people to provide support for the elderly who are in need of care.

Our understanding of these trends as they apply to the society at large has made it possible for us to recognize their manifestation in the population of mentally retarded persons.

Another important point is that the field of mental retardation has "come of age." Despite the fact that mental retardation is the single largest category of lifelong handicaps, professionals in our field spent literally decades focused almost exclusively on the study of and care for children with disabilities. Mentally retarded persons were viewed as and often treated like children even in adulthood. It was not until the early 1970s that adults with mental retardation became the focus of a substantial amount of concern. The need for age-appropriate services for mentally retarded adults is now commonly recognized by professionals in the field. It is not surprising that 15 years after the time when the field expanded its vision to include adulthood, we are now straining our eyes to examine the next stage, namely old age.

In this context, the development of programs specifically geared towards meeting the needs of mentally retarded elders extends the continuum of services for this population. The concept of continuum of services has provided an important framework for defining the range or types of programs needed to increase the skills and capacity for independence among mentally retarded persons. Until recently, however, the continuum did not include a consideration of the needs of elderly persons. As the chapters in this monograph describe, these needs are now being addressed by a sizable number of programs across the country.

At the present time, there are three basic service options for elderly persons with mental retardation. These are:

1. including elderly mentally retarded persons in programs for younger mentally retarded adults (the *age integration option*);
2. including elderly mentally retarded persons in programs for the general elderly population (the *generic services integration option*); and
3. developing specialized services for elderly mentally retarded persons (the *specialized service option*).

THE AGE
INTEGRATION OPTION

The most common approach to providing services to elderly mentally retarded persons is to include them in programs serving mentally retarded adults of all ages. According to research conducted at the University of Minnesota's Center for Residential and Community Services, in 1982 nearly 25% of all mentally retarded persons served in community residences in the U.S. were between the ages of 40 and 62 and another 5% were aged 63 and over (Hauber, Rotegard, & Bruininks, 1985). They also reported an almost 4% increase between 1978 and 1982 in the percentage of residents between the ages of 40 and 62. These data suggest that residents are "aging in place."

One important reason for the dominance of the age integration option is that there is good evidence to suggest that elderly mentally retarded service recipients *as a group* do not necessarily function at a lower level than younger mentally retarded persons because of the differential composition of the older and younger cohorts (discussed in more detail in Chapter 2). Thus, it is possible to maintain or integrate some aging mentally retarded persons into programs for younger mentally retarded adults without substantially modifying the services offered or the expectations made of the clients. In this context, age alone has not been a barrier to service integration.

THE GENERIC SERVICES
INTEGRATION OPTION

This service option integrates elderly mentally retarded persons in services designed for the general (i.e., nonretarded) elderly population. This is probably the least commonly used option for a mentally retarded person's *day* program but more commonly used option for *residential* programs. With respect to residential services, a commonly utilized generic service program is the nursing home that serves both retarded and elderly persons. Data from the 1977 National Nursing Home Survey indicated that approximately 42,000 persons whose primary diagnosis was mental retardation lived in nursing homes (Lakin, 1985). Over half of these residents were age 55 or older.

While Seltzer and Wells (1986) reported that there are generic senior citizen programs that accept mentally retarded clients, and indeed, have positive experiences to report, the absolute number of mentally retarded persons involved in such programs nationwide is estimated to be very small. The feasibility and appropriateness of integrating elderly mentally retarded persons into generic senior citizen programs is largely a function of the extent to which the elderly mentally retarded and the elderly nonretarded participants share common characteristics and needs. High functioning elderly mentally retarded persons may be excellent candidates for mainstreaming into generic senior citizen programs. Such individuals generally compare favorably with nonretarded elderly persons who may have serious chronic illnesses and cognitive and functional limitations. Thus, having mental retardation alone may not be a barrier to utilization of generic services.

THE SPECIALIZED
SERVICE OPTION

In this option, special services are developed for elderly persons with mental retardation in order to respond to their special needs. Programmatic features characteristic of such services include a slower pace, more opportunities for personal choice, more recreational and leisure time activities, and an increased attention to clients' health needs. The National Survey of Programs Serving Elderly Mentally Retarded Persons was designed to collect in-depth information about the specialized service option.

PURPOSE OF THE
NATIONAL SURVEY

The purpose of the National Survey of Programs Serving Elderly Mentally Retarded Persons was to identify and describe community and institutionally based programs in which at least 50% of the mentally retarded persons served were age 55 and over. Our goal was to identify programs with a "critical mass" of elderly mentally retarded persons.

The survey was designed to address the following questions:

1. What is the national distribution of programs serving elderly mentally retarded persons? What factors contribute to the variability among states in their development of such programs?
2. To what extent are programs serving elderly mentally retarded persons available in community as compared with institutional settings? Given the well documented shift in the age distribution within institutional facilities, are community-based services lagging behind or are they ahead of what is available in public residential facilities?
3. What are the administrative and management characteristics of these programs? Are they sponsored by multiprogram agencies or are they primarily demonstration projects, the lifespans of which are uncertain?
4. What are the characteristics of the mentally retarded persons served in these programs?
5. What is the range of services provided by these programs?
6. What types of staff are employed in these programs and to what extent are specialized skills or training needed and/or available?

7. What special or unique problems and challenges confront programs in serving elderly mentally retarded persons?

8. To what extent have programs serving elderly mentally retarded persons accessed generic senior centers on behalf of their clients?

9. To what extent have mentally retarded people "retired" from day programs that may no longer meet their motivational, energy, or interest levels? What are the characteristics of innovative or exemplary retirement options?

10. What recommendations do staff from existing programs have for other programs or agencies interested in developing programs for elderly mentally retarded persons? What do staff from existing programs wish they had known prior to serving this population?

The National Survey was not designed as an evaluation study—either of discrete programs or of statewide activity. No attempt was made to measure the extent to which programs met their specified goals, improved the quality of life of the clients they served, or were cost-effective service models. Rather, the research was designed to be an exploratory and descriptive investigation into the range, styles, and contexts in which elderly mentally retarded persons received residential and day services in the United States.

The results of the National Survey provide answers to many basic questions about the distribution and characteristics of, and the challenges faced by, programs serving elderly mentally retarded persons. This information is particularly critical in order to aid the design and conduct of subsequent studies that address specific types of policy, programmatic, and client outcomes. In addition, the development of this baseline knowledge may aid in the design and creation of services for elders with mental retardation.

ORGANIZATION OF
THE VOLUME

The monograph is organized in three sections. Section I sets the context for the project by providing a review of the literature on aging and mental retardation (Chapter 2) and by presenting the methods and procedures by which the study was conducted (Chapter 3).

Section II presents the results of the analyses. It begins with a description of the national distribution and development of programs for elderly mentally retarded persons (Chapter 4). Chapters 5 and 6 describe community-based residential and day programs, while Chapter 7 discusses institutionally based programs. Chapter 8 presents a detailed description of six comprehensive residential and day programs that provide long term care for elderly mentally retarded persons.

Section III includes three chapters that focus on broad issues facing the continued growth of programs serving elderly mentally retarded persons. The issues discussed—the use of generic senior centers (Chapter 9), retirement options (Chapter 10), and the research, service, and policy needs of the field (Chapter 11)—are based both on the empirical results of the National Survey and on the literature from the fields of gerontology and mental retardation.

Chapter 2

Characteristics of Elderly Mentally Retarded Persons
A Review of the Literature

As Baird and Sadovnick (1985) noted, "mental retardation is the single largest catergory of life-long handicaps affecting populations in 'developed' countries" (p. 323). However, researchers, policy analysts, and service providers have traditionally focused their attention on mentally retarded children, adolescents, and young adults, while the characteristics and needs of persons in middle and old age are largely undocumented and poorly understood.

The literature on the aging process for mentally retarded persons is therefore limited. However, a flurry of publications have appeared during the past few years that contain a substantial amount of information that informed the conceptualization and orientation of the National Survey. This chapter summarizes past research on aging and mental retardation with respect to the following three questions:

1. What is the best definition of *old age* for this population?
2. How many mentally retarded persons are currently considered to be elderly?
3. What are the characteristics of mentally retarded persons who have reached old age?

Literature about the service needs of elderly mentally retarded persons will be discussed in Chapters 5 through 8. In the discussion that follows, we draw upon literature on aging in mentally retarded persons and upon relevant research from the field of gerontology to enrich our examination of the questions listed above.

WHAT IS THE BEST DEFINITION OF *OLD AGE* FOR THIS POPULATION?

A prerequisite for effective planning and service delivery for any group is the development of a reliable and valid definition of the population of concern. An examination of the gerontological literature reveals the complexity of developing a valid definition of old age for the general (i.e., non-mentally retarded) population. This task has proven to be particularly difficult with respect to older persons with mental retardation.

Most gerontologists have defined old age in years. Common ages used to demarcate the onset of old age include 60, 62, 65, and 72 (Siegel, 1980). Some gerontologists (e.g., Streib, 1983) differentiate the "young old" (ages 65–74) and the "old-old" (ages 75 +), although other interval limits have also been used to divide the elderly into two age groups.

Federal policies have defined old age in various ways. For example, whereas under the Older Americans Act age 60 has been designated as the age basis on which service eligibility is determined, the Social Security Administration uses age 65 as the age criterion at which a host of income and medical supports become available.

Alternative models for the definition of aging and old age also have been proposed in the gerontological literature. Siegel (1980) suggested that old age could be defined as the period of life beginning at an arbitrarily chosen fixed number of years before the expected time of death for a particular subgroup of the population. For example, if the average life expectancy for men is 72 years and for women 78, and if the last 10 years of life were to be considered to be old age, this stage would begin at age 62 for men and at age 68 for women.

There are also functionally based definitions of old age. For example, Eisdorfer (1983) identified four stages in life: children and youth in whom society invests resources in anticipation of future benefit; adult workers (paid and unpaid) who generate the goods and services utilized by the entire society; healthy persons who have retired from paid employment but who are not functionally dependent upon others; and frail individuals who cannot function independently. Yet another approach to the definition of aging was summarized by Birren (1959), who conceptualized three components of aging: biological aging, which is an individual's capacity for survival; psychological aging, which consist of changes in a person's adaptive capacities; and social aging, which is the extent to which an individual fulfills the expected social and cultural roles.

Many difficulties arise in the application of these alternative definitional models to mentally retarded persons. Siegel's (1980) model of defining old age as the last n years before a subgroup's expected age of death cannot be easily applied to mentally retarded persons in light of both the lack of good data about true life expectancy for this population (unconfounded by factors such as the quality of health care received throughout the life span) and the astounding progress that has been made in extending the length of life for various subgroups of mentally retarded persons (e.g., individuals with Down syndrome). Eisdorfer's (1983) model is also inappropriate because many moderately and severely retarded adults younger than 55 or 60 years of age function in Eisdorfer's categories 3 and 4 (the categories he designated as elderly). In this regard, the absence of a high correlation between chronological age and functional abilities has long been recognized as a defining characteristic of mental retardation.

Similarly, in Birren's model, limitations in psychological and social performance, viewed as *functional aging*, both contain elements of the American Association on Mental Retardation's definition of adaptive behavior (Grossman, 1983), one of the three criteria used to define mental retardation. A lack of conceptual clarity would exist if a study used the same criteria to define both old age and mental retardation.

The difficulty in applying these alternative conceptualizations of aging to mentally retarded persons illustrates why most literature on aging and mental retardation has used a chronological definition of old age. A recent survey of state councils on developmental disabilities and state units on aging found an age range of 55 to 65 years used to identify older persons with mental retardation (Janicki, Ackerman, & Jacobson, 1985). Some policy analysts have suggested that the field of mental retardation should conform to the age criterion embodied in the Older Americans Act of 1965 (PL 89–73, as amended), which specifies age 60 as the lower age limit of eligibility for services (Janicki, Knox, & Jacobson, 1985). However, at the present time there is no consensus among professionals in the field of mental retardation as to whether age 60 or some older or younger age should be defined for this population. As shown in Table 2-1, the published literature contains research reports, policy and planning documents, and practice descriptions that variously define the onset of old age for mentally retarded persons at anywhere from 40 to 75.

Reasons for the widely varying lower age limits for the definition of old age in the population of mentally retarded persons include evidence that: mentally retarded persons begin to decline in behavioral capacities during their 50s (Puccio, Janicki, Otis, & Rettig, 1983); there is an increased incidence and earlier onset of Alzheimer's Disease among persons with Down syndrome (Lott & Lai, 1982; Miniszek, 1983); and retarded persons have a shorter average lifespan than the general population (Eyman, Grossman, Tarjan, & Miller, 1987; Richards, 1976; Tarjan, Wright, Eyman, and Keeran, 1973). However, due to the heterogeneous nature of the population with mental retardation, each of these three trends is applicable to some population subgroups but not to all mentally retarded persons. Specifically, persons whose retardation is mild or moderate have very different social, educational, medical, and functional characteristics and service histories from those whose retarda-

TABLE 2-1

Cutoff Points Used in the Literature on Aging and Mental Retardation

AGE	CITATION
40	Dy, Strain, Fullerton, & Stowitschek, 1981 Hauber, Rotegard, & Bruininks, 1985 ("older adults") Kriger, 1975, 1976 Wood, 1979
45	Dubrow, 1967 Janicki & Jacobson, 1984a Reid & Aungle, 1974 Sherman, Frenkel, & Newman, 1984
50	Anglin, 1981 Baker, Seltzer, & Seltzer, 1977 Mueller & Porter, 1969 Talkington & Chiovaro, 1969
53	Janicki & MacEachron, 1984 ("late middle aged") Sutton, 1983 ("late middle aged")
55	Hamilton & Segal, 1975 Krauss & Seltzer, 1984 Kultgen, Rinck, Calkins, & Intagliata, 1986 Neuman, 1981 Puccio, Janicki, Otis, & Rettig, 1983 ("aging") Richards & Siddiqui, 1980 Segal, 1977 Seltzer, Seltzer, & Sherwood, 1982
60	Cotton, Purzycki, Cowart, & Merritt, 1983 Cotton, Sison, & Starr, 1981 Keiter, 1979 Mather, 1981 O'Connor, Justice, & Warren, 1970
63	Hauber, Rotegard, & Bruininks, 1985 ("elderly adults") Janicki & MacEachron, 1984 ("aging") Sutton, 1983 ("aging")
65	Baroff, 1982
70	Synder & Woolner, 1974
73	Janicki & MacEachron, 1984 ("aged") Sutton, 1983 ("aged")
75	Puccio, Janicki, Otis, & Rettig, 1983 ("aged")

tion is classified as severe or profound (Best-Sigford, Bruininks, Lakin, Hill, & Heal, 1982; Lakin, Krantz, Bruininks, Clumpner, & Hill, 1982) and may age in different ways with respect to each of the three trends noted above. Similarly, it is commonly noted that mentally retarded persons who are without additional physical handicaps differ in many respects from those who have some organic basis for their retardation, who are generally more severely retarded and have multiple handicaps (Grossman, 1983; Zigler, Balla and Hodapp, 1984). The life expectancy and aging process for these two groups probably differ substantially, further diminishing the validity of viewing the aging process among retarded persons as a unitary phenomenon.

In designing the National Survey, the gerontological and mental retardation literatures on the definition of old age were reviewed. Age 55 was selected for our study as the lower limit of the onset of old age among the mentally retarded persons in the programs that were studied. The use of any age cutoff is arbitrary and poses a risk of misclassification of individuals. We had no reasonable method for estimating the extent to which age 55 or any other age cutoff incorrectly classified persons as "elderly," given their individual levels of functioning and age. We weighed the magnitude of the risks of two types of misclassification, given a series of potential cutoff points. The use of age 55 probably resulted in the inclusion of some individuals who, on the basis of their current physical, psychological, and social abilities, would not be considered "elderly" in any functional sense of the word. At the same time, the use of age 55 excluded younger individuals who have already exhibited signs of premature aging (e.g., individuals with Down syndrome). While these types of inappropriate classifications will be present with the use of any chronologically based definition of aging, in our judgment age 55 best minimized the frequency of both of these errors in classification.

HOW MANY MENTALLY RETARDED PERSONS ARE CURRENTLY CONSIDERED TO BE ELDERLY?

Estimates (based on the 1980 census) of the number of persons with mental retardation aged 55 and over range from 1,417,320 (based on a 3% mental retardation prevalence rate) to 472,440 (based on a 1% prevalence rate). However, only 196,000 mentally retarded persons are currently known to receive state supported mental retardation services (Jacobson, Sutton, & Janicki, 1985).

Estimates of the number of elderly mentally retarded persons are needed by service planners and budget analysts for long range planning. However, it may be invalid to use estimates based on the number of known service recipients for future planning purposes because many persons who are mentally retarded and over age 55 are not currently known to the formal service system. It has been suggested, for example, that as many as 40% of the estimated number of elderly mentally retarded persons are not known to formal service delivery systems (Krauss, 1986). To further illustrate this point, in Edgerton's most recent follow-up study (Edgerton, Bollinger, & Herr, 1984), not a single member of the sample (all but one of whom were over age 50) was receiving any service from the formal mental retardation service network; thus, all would likely have been omitted from estimates of the prevalence of old age among mentally retarded persons.

A direct epidemiological study of this population has not yet been conducted and thus accurate counts are not available. It is not possible to use epidemiological data collected about mentally retarded children or young adults to make projections about this population in old age because surviving members of any cohort differ markedly from the birth cohort's characteristics. In the mental retardation population, the nonrepresentativeness of surviving individuals is attributable to genetic, metabolic, and physical disorders, birth traumas, and other disabilities associated with a shorter lifespan. Thus, epidemiological and descriptive data about aging mentally retarded persons are needed in order to make valid estimates for research, planning, and service provision.

WHAT ARE THE CHARACTERISTICS OF ELDERLY MENTALLY RETARDED PERSONS?

Demographic Characteristics

Previous studies of aging and mental retardation have often included demographic descriptions of their samples with respect to age, sex, and level of retardation. These data are presented in Table 2-2. Because of the idiosyncratic procedures with which most of these samples were selected, it is difficult to generalize population characteristics from the data presented in Table 2-2. However, a number of trends and relationships can be detected.

- *The percentage of females seems to rise with advancing age.* As shown in the Janicki and MacEachron (1984) and the Sutton (1983) studies, there is at least a 10 percentage point difference between the proportion of females in the youngest cohort (aged 53 to 62) and the oldest cohort (aged 73 and older). This positive relationship between age and percentage of females mirrors the longer life expectancy of women as compared with men characteristic of the population in general. Data from the 1980 US census are illustrative of this trend. The proportions of the total US population that are female for those aged 55–64, 65–74, 75–84, and 85 and older are 53%, 57%, 63%, and 70%, respectively. Thus, the "greying" of the population with mental retardation, as in the general population, carries with it a shift in the ratio of males to females.

TABLE 2-2

Demographic Characteristics of Elderly Mentally Retarded Persons

STUDY	AGE RANGE	AGE MEAN	SEX % FEMALE	MEAN IQ	LEVEL OF RETARDATION % MILD/ MODERATE	LEVEL OF RETARDATION % SEVERE/ PROFOUND
Baker, Seltzer, & Seltzer, 1977	50+	59	66			
Carsrud & Carsrud, 1983		61	0	32		
Cotton, Purzycki, Cowart, & Merritt, 1983	60–87	69				
Cotton, Sison, & Starr, 1981			32			
Edgerton, Bollinger, & Herr, 1984	47–68	56	47	62		
Hauber, Rotegard, & Bruininks, 1985						
a) community-based facilities	40–62	45			69	31
	63+	50			88	12
b) public residential facilities	40–62	47			30	70
	63+	64			38	62
Janicki & Jacobson, 1984b	50–99					
Janicki & Jacobson, 1986b	45–94				46	53
Janicki & MacEachron, 1984	53–62		48		41	51
	63–72		51		42	48
	73+		61		38	50
Krauss & Seltzer, 1986	55–91	63	49			
Reid & Aungle, 1974	45+		59		80	20
Seltzer, Seltzer, & Sherwood, 1982	55+	64	64	49		
Sherman, Frenkel, & Newman, 1984	46–92	63	58		67	33
Snyder & Woolner, 1974	70–88	75				
Sutton, 1983	53–62		49		58	42
	63–72		53		60	40
	73+		60		53	47
Wood, 1979	41+		40		85	10

- *On the basis of cross-sectional data, level of retardation does not seem to decline with advancing age.* We know that subgroups of the population show marked declines in their intellectual capacities as they age (e.g., persons with Down syndrome). However, in heterogeneous groups of mentally retarded persons, no such trend is apparent. The data from the Janicki & MacEachron (1984) and Sutton (1983) studies illustrate this point. Our previous research has suggested that the cognitive abilities of mentally retarded persons aged 55 to 74 do not differ significantly from those of mentally retarded persons over age 75 (Krauss & Seltzer, 1986). However, longitudinal analyses are needed to separate cohort effects from true maturational changes (Seltzer, 1985).

- *The samples studied contained very old persons.* While a number of studies included individuals as young as their 40s (e.g., Janicki & Jacobson, 1984a; Sherman et al., 1984; Wood, 1979), the average ages of sample members (when the mean was reported) were generally over 60 and the oldest sample members (when the upper end of the range was reported) were over 85. In early literature on aging and mental retardation, middle-aged adults were often the focus of study, while the more recent research summarized in Table 2-2 suggests that individuals who would commonly be seen as elderly comprise the study groups.

The National Survey of Programs Serving Elderly Mentally Retarded Persons will supplement demographic data available from previous research by reporting the age distribution, sex, and level of retardation of persons over the age of 55 who are served by age-specialized residential and day programs in institutional and community-based settings. The extent to which different types of programs include special subgroups of the elderly mentally retarded population (e.g., the "old old", the severely and profoundly retarded) will also be examined from the National Survey data set.

Health and Functional Abilities

While it is generally assumed that older mentally retarded adults have more health impairments and functional limitations than younger adults, only a few studies have reported data about these issues and these have produced conflicting findings. Janicki and MacEachron (1984) found that elderly mentally retarded persons received more medical services than younger adult sample members, suggesting that the elderly had more serious medical needs. In a further analysis of these data, Janicki and Jacobson (1986b) reported that the older the age cohort, the greater the percentage of elderly mentally retarded persons who had chronic diseases and the greater the number of different medical conditions manifested by the cohort members. In contrast, Seltzer, Seltzer, and Sherwood (1982) found that elderly and younger adult sample members did not differ in number of health problems. Similarly, Krauss and Seltzer (1986) reported that the elderly did not differ from younger mentally retarded adults in medical impairments or medical services received, but the elderly had more sensory impairments. Kaiser, Montague, Wold, Maune, and Pattison (1981) reported an increased percentage of individuals with impaired hearing associated with advancing age among a sample of adults with Down syndrome. A similar association between age and hearing loss among adults with Down syndrome was reported by Brooks, Wooley, and Kanjilal (1972).

Regarding functional limitations, Seltzer et al. (1982) reported that the elderly were more functionally impaired than the younger group studied, while Krauss and Seltzer (1986) found that the younger adult group was more functionally impaired than the elderly group. In contrast with these two cross-sectional studies, Silverstein, Herbs, Nasuta, and White (1986) reported in a longitudinal study that the functional abilities of institutionalized persons with Down syndrome and mentally retarded persons with other diagnoses declined with advancing age. Janicki and Jacobson (1986b) presented a more fine grained cross-sectional analysis of age-related differences in functional abilities among their aging cohorts. Among mildly and moderately retarded persons, declining abilities in motoric skills were observed at about age 50, while declining cognitive skills were observed in the aged 70 to 74 cohort. Among severely and profoundly retarded persons, declines in motoric and cognitive skills were not evident until after age 70. This surprising finding may be attributable to a mortality rate higher in the severely and profoundly retarded cohort than in the mildly and moderately retarded cohort.

Clearly, more research is needed to fully describe the health and functional characteristics of mentally retarded persons in old age. It is possible that the inconsistencies in findings reported in these studies are attributable to a somewhat unique subgroup of the population with mental retardation being included in each study and to the differences between longitudinal and cross-sectional designs. The use of probability sampling methods and longitudinal designs in future research are therefore important methodological considerations.

The National Survey will supplement available data on the health and functional abilities of elderly mentally retarded persons by providing descriptive information about the health and functional impairments of clients served in the programs studied and by examining differences in the characteristics of clients served among program types.

Family Relationships

In the general population, it is the informal support system—primarily the family—that provides the bulk of services for elderly persons (Brody, 1979; Silverman & Brahce, 1979). Because of the efforts of family members, as many as 60% of the extremely impaired elderly live outside of institutions (Shanas & Sussman, 1981) and fully 80% of their service needs are met by the informal support system (Hooyman, 1983). In most cases, support is provided by a spouse or by adult daughters, daughters-in-law, or sons.

Unlike most elderly, aging mentally retarded persons generally do not have children or a spouse on whom they can depend for support. In some cases, there are very old parents who still provide some support to the already elderly retarded person. However, in most cases mentally retarded persons' family network consists of siblings and the children of siblings. No research has been conducted on changes in the quality of sibling relationships over the full life cycle in families with a mentally retarded child, although some data on adult siblings are available (Cleveland & Miller, 1977; Zetlin, 1986). Past research on families, however, has suggested that siblings of retarded children may be at risk for adjustment problems that may impair their ability to provide informal support in adulthood and old age (Crnic, Friedrich, & Greenberg, 1983; Intagliata & Doyle, 1984; Zetlin, 1986).

As in the general population, the informal support system of aging mentally retarded persons includes friends as well as family. It is possible that the role of friends might be even more important for elderly mentally retarded persons, given their more limited network of relatives in this stage of life (Kultgen, Rinck, Calkins, & Intagliata, 1986). Edgerton (1967) conceptualized and documented the role played by benefactor in the lives of the formerly institutionalized adults he studied. Were it not for these benefactors, many of the study group would have been at risk for reinstitutionalization. Although no research has specifically examined the patterns of friendships among older mentally retarded persons, in previous studies of patterns of affiliation among heterogeneous age groups of mentally retarded adults, age has been found to be associated with less affiliative and social behavior (Berkson & Romer, 1980; Landesman-Dwyer, Berkson, & Romer, 1979; Landesman-Dwyer, Sackett, & Kleinman, 1980; Romer & Berkson, 1980a, 1980b, 1981).

Past research is available regarding the extent to which elderly mentally retarded persons live with their families. These studies are summarized in Table 2-3. One finding common to these studies was that the percentage of elderly persons who lived with their families was lower in older cohorts. Rowitz (1980) noted that while just over 30% of the California clients he studied between the ages of 50 and 59 lived with their families, this number dropped to 4% in the 60 to 80 year old group, and no individual over the age of 80 lived with a relative. Of the studies summarized in Table 2-3, Rowitz's data reflect the highest rates of elderly persons living with family members. The lowest rates were reported by Krauss and Seltzer (1986), who found that of those who received state supported services in Massachusetts, slightly under 2% of those between the ages of 55 and 74 and not one person over the age of 75 lived with relatives. No data are currently available regarding the frequency of family contact among older mentally retarded persons who do not live with relatives.

In sum, little is known about the pattern of family relationships and

TABLE 2-3

Percentages of Older Mentally Retarded Persons Who Live with Family

AUTHOR AND GEOGRAPHIC LOCATION OF SAMPLE	AGE RANGE	PERCENT LIVING WITH FAMILY			
Best-Sigford, Bruininks, Lakin, Hill, & Heal (1982) (nationwide)	40–63	12.0			
	64+	0.0			
Janicki & MacEachron (1984) (New York)	52–62	7.0			
	63–72	3.0			
	73+	1.0			
Krauss & Seltzer (1986) (Massachusetts)	55–74	1.8			
	75+	0.0			
Rowitz (1980) (California)	50–59	31.2			
	60–80	4.4			
	81+	0.0			
Seltzer & Seltzer (1978) (Massachusetts)	55+	8.0			
Sutton (1983) (California)	53–62	17.3			
	63–72	11.1			
	73+	6.5			
		MI	MOD	SEV	PRO
Meyers, Borthwick, & Eyman (1985) (California)	50–54	27	25	17	2
	55–59	25	20	10	2
	60–64	12	8	8	1
	65+	12	8	8	1

supports for mentally retarded persons in old age. However, it can be inferred from past research on the general elderly population that the maintenance of some contact with family members is very important with respect to the quality of life of aging mentally retarded persons. For this reason, research that attempts to identify factors predictive of the maintenance of family ties is needed.

While the National Survey was essentially a study of the formal service system, some information about the informal support system—families, in particular—was collected. For example, the proportion of clients who lived with their families prior to their current living arrangement will be reported for residential programs, as will the proportion of day program clients who currently live with their families. In addition, strategies that programs have used to maintain and strengthen relationships between clients and family members will be examined.

Differences Between Elderly and Younger Mentally Retarded Adults

It is commonly assumed that elderly mentally retarded persons have needs that are different from those of younger retarded adults (Anglin,

1981; DiGiovanni, 1978; Segal, 1977; Sweeney & Wilson, 1979). This argument is consistent with evidence that the health, functional abilities, and availability of informal supports of the general population decline with advancing age (Kart, Metress & Metress, 1978; Lowenthal & Robinson, 1976; Neugarten, 1982).

The extent to which these age-related differences are characteristic of mentally retarded persons has been directly examined in only a few studies, which have produced conflicting findings. While Edgerton et al. (1984), based on a longitudinal study, reported an improved quality of life associated with advancing age, other studies using cross-sectional designs have found that elderly persons have more health problems and receive fewer services than younger mentally retarded adults (Janicki & MacEachron, 1984; Krauss & Seltzer, 1986). These conflicting findings are attributable at least in part to differences in the characteristics of the samples across studies (e.g., mildly retarded vs. all levels of retardation and to different research methodologies used (qualitative vs. quantitative).

In attempting to determine whether elderly and younger adult mentally retarded persons have different service needs, it is necessary to be cautious about assuming that differences between older and younger cohorts are caused by the maturational effects of aging. In fact, such differences might be attributable to a host of factors that could affect older cohorts but not younger groups or vice versa. These include changes in the eligibility criteria for state-supported mental retardation services that have occurred during this century and the shorter life span characteristic of severely and profoundly retarded persons. These two factors alone would cause older cohorts to seem to be less seriously retarded than younger cohorts because older cohorts include "borderline" mentally retarded persons who would not be so labelled today and who are thus not included in younger cohorts and because younger cohorts contain severely and profoundly retarded persons who are not expected to live to old age and who are thus not included in older cohorts.

Further research, preferably utilizing longitudinal design, is needed to determine the magnitude and nature of age-related differences among mentally retarded persons. For planning purposes, this knowledge would be useful in assessing the need for age-specialized versus age-integrated mental retardation services. Small differences between younger adults and elderly mentally retarded persons would argue for age-integrated mental retardation services, whereas larger differences would argue for age-specialized mental retardation services.

The National Survey collected extensive information about programs in which all clients were over age 55 and programs in which more than half but not all clients were over age 55. These data will illustrate the range of service options that currently exist for elderly mentally retarded persons.

Differences Between Elderly Mentally Retarded and Nonretarded Persons

A related issue pertains to the feasibility of including aging mentally retarded persons in services designed for the nonretarded elderly population. While Dybwad (1962) raised this issue over 20 years ago, only a few studies have been conducted to assess the degree of difference between these two groups.

In two studies, elderly mentally retarded persons were found to deteriorate more in sensory and functional abilities than did the nonretarded elders with whom they were compared. Callison, Armstrong, Elam, Cannon, Paisley, and Himwich (1971) compared elderly mentally retarded, elderly schizophrenic, and elderly nondisabled persons with respect to changes over time in their visual ability, hearing, and grip strength. While all groups were found to deteriorate over time in these three areas, the mentally retarded elderly deteriorated the most in vision and hearing. Sherwood and Morris (1983) also studied mentally retarded, mentally ill, and elderly persons in an evaluation of the Pennsylvania Domiciliary Care Program. The three client groups were found to respond similarly to placement in a domiciliary care home in many respects, with the exception that the mentally retarded clients deteriorated in functional abilities over time while the other two groups did not.

A different pattern of findings was reported by Cotton, Sison, and Starr (1981), who compared elderly mentally retarded residents of a public mental retardation facility with nonretarded elderly residents of an Intermediate Care Facility (ICF), and nonretarded elderly persons who lived in the community. While the nonretarded elderly persons who lived in the community were found to be superior in functioning to the other two groups, the elderly retarded subjects were found to function at a higher level than did the elderly ICF group in all domains except for communication.

These studies highlight the fact that different degrees of similarity and difference between elderly retarded and elderly nonretarded persons will be found depending upon the subgroup of each population that is studied. In future research, it may be productive to compare elderly retarded and elderly nonretarded persons who have been closely matched on age, health status, and current residential arrangement to determine the feasibility of integrating such groups for service delivery.

The National Survey included some generic senior programs in which mentally retarded clients were served along with other elderly persons. Examination of the difficulties that such programs have encountered as they attempted to integrate mentally retarded elders will provide information about the feasibility of such integration efforts. Also, data about the utilization of generic senior centers by all programs included in the National Survey will provide some preliminary information about the extent and success of attempts to access such services for mentally retarded elders.

CONCLUSIONS

The research literature on the characteristics of elderly mentally retarded persons, though relatively small in size and recent in origin, suggests a number of important conclusions that define the current context for programs serving elderly mentally retarded persons. First, the population of elders with mental retardation is very heterogeneous with respect to age, health, functional abilities, cognitive abilities, and informal supports. This level of heterogeneity suggests that a wide variety of services will be needed to meet the needs of various subgroups of this population. No single model of service delivery is likely to be applicable to all potential service recipients.

Second, the number of elderly mentally retarded persons in the US has increased and will continue to increase in the foreseeable future. However, precise estimates of size of this group are not yet available because of two factors: the lack of an agreed upon definition of the lower age limit of this stage of life, and the focus of epidemiological studies on aging service recipients rather than on both served and unserved elderly mentally retarded persons. Thus, service planners and policy analysts will be hampered in their long range planning efforts until such issues are resolved and better estimates become available.

Third, inconsistencies in findings from study to study are attributable, at least in part, to differences between cross-sectional and longitudinal studies. In cross-sectional studies, differences between cohorts may or may not be indicative of the effects of aging because generational differences confound aging effects. In longitudinal studies, the effects of loss of sample members caused by dropping out or death may confound our understanding of the effects of aging. Thus, future studies on age-related trends in the population of elderly mentally retarded persons must attend to these methodological concerns if they are to shed increasing light on as yet unanswered substantive questions.

The National Survey of Programs Serving Elderly Mentally Retarded persons addressed yet another gap in the current literature, namely on analysis of the continuum of specialized residential and day programs that currently serve elderly mentally retarded persons. Because the continuum of services has only recently been extended to serve mentally retarded persons in old age, our nationwide descriptive study was conducted in order to take stock of the current range of program options for this segment of the population with mental retardation.

Chapter 3

Study Methods and Procedures

The National Survey was conducted in four phases. Phase I, Study Conceptualization, produced a designation of an age cutoff for defining the elderly mentally retarded population (for the reasons described in Chapter 2) and a set of programmatic criteria for inclusion in the study (described below). Phase II, Sample Selection, consisted of formulating operational definitions of the range of programs to be surveyed, determining methods by which such programs could be identified, obtaining lists of programs, and screening potentially eligible programs to yield the study sample. Phase III, Data Collection, involved the conduct of extensive telephone interviews investigating all identified programs that met the study criteria. The methods and procedures for completing these phases are described in this chapter. The results of Phase IV, Data Analysis, are presented in the remaining chapters of the monograph.

PHASE I: CONCEPTUALIZATION OF THE PROJECT

As discussed in Chapter 2, a key decision for the study was the designation of age 55 as the minimum age for defining the target population. A second major task was to define the types of programs to be included. We were interested in surveying institutional and community-based residential and day programs, including nonvocationally oriented social and recreational programs. We were further interested in surveying programs that because of either their design or the demographic characteristics of their clients had a substantial percentage of mentally retarded clients in the 55 and older age range.

In order to operationalize these goals, the following program criteria were developed:

(1) At least 50% of the mentally retarded persons served in the program were age 55 or over.

(2) The program served at last two mentally retarded persons aged 55 and over.

(3) If the program served both mentally retarded and other types of clients (for example, nonhandicapped elderly), at least 10% of the

total clients served in the program must be mentally retarded. if the program met this criterion, then the "50% rule" (#1 above) was applied to the number of mentally retarded persons served.

(4) The program was in operation as of or before January 1, 1985.

As with the choice of an age cutoff, the decision to restrict our sample to programs in which a minimum of 50% of the mentally retarded clients served were age 55 or over was somewhat arbitrary. Our intent was to include programs in which a majority of the clients were in their older years. The second criterion, which limited sampled programs to those with at least two mentally retarded persons aged 55 or over, was intended to exclude very small programs such as foster homes in which there were two mentally retarded persons, only one of whom was over age 55. The third criterion, which required that at least 10% of the clients served in a program were mentally retarded, excluded programs in which only a small number of mentally retarded persons participated as compared with the size of the nonretarded group served.

PHASE II: SAMPLE
SELECTION PROCEDURES

Operational Definitions

The next issue faced was identifying potential programs to be surveyed. We defined the pool of institutional programs from which our survey would draw as those facilities listed in the Directory of Public Residential Facilities for the Mentally Retarded prepared by the National Association of Superintendents of Public Residential Facilities for the Mentally Retarded (1984). These facilities all fit the definition of a "living quarter which provided 24-hour, 7 days a week responsibility for room, board and supervision of mentally retarded persons" as used in the University of Minnesota's Developmental Disabilities Project on Residential Services and Community Adjustment (Hauber, Bruininks, Hill, Lakin & White, 1984, p. 3).

Our definition of a community-based residential program was a regulated facility providing room, board, and some degree of protective oversight (i.e., some service beyond room and board and basic maintenance of laundry) to mentally retarded persons. This definition is comparable to that used by other studies of community-based residential programs (Hauber, Bruininks, Hill, Lakin, & White, 1984; Sherwood & Seltzer, 1981). We specifically excluded nursing homes and family homes from the study.

Our definition of community-based day programs was a regulated program or facility providing recreational, pre-vocational, vocational, leisure, or social activities.

Identifying and Screening Potential Programs

Developing a process for identifying an efficient pool from which to sample community-based residential and day programs posed a difficult challenge. We knew that many of the programs that would meet our criteria had begun operation very recently and that in some instances their special focus on serving elderly mentally retarded persons would not be known to state regulatory agencies. We also determined that surveying the approximately 15,633 community-based residential facilities identified by the University of Minnesota's project on residential services would be prohibitively costly and would miss those programs that had begun operation after June 1982 (Hauber, Bruininks, Hill, Lakin, & White, 1984). Given the presumption that many of the programs of interest to the present study were of recent origin, we developed a multistage process for identifying relevant sampling pools from which to select programs.

We cast a wide net in publicizing the National Survey and in developing our own lists of programs, agencies, and administrators to contact. First, we obtained the endorsements for the project from the American Association on Mental Retardation and from the National Association of Superintendents of Public Mental Retardation Facilities. These letters of endorsement were included in all of the mailings described below. Second, we used the following procedures for identifying programs:

(1) Commissioners or directors of state departments of mental retardation, mental health, and aging in each of the 50 states and the District of Columbia were contacted and asked to identify programs known to them that served elderly mentally retarded persons.

(2) The executive directors of all state chapters of the Association for Retarded Citizens (ARCs) were contacted and asked to identify relevant programs known to them and to include a description of our study (provided to them) in their state and local mailings.

(3) The Association for Retarded Citizens-U.S. included a description of the National Survey and a request that potentially relevant

programs contact the project in a national mailing to approximately 2,500 individuals, groups, and agencies.

(4) Project descriptions were published in approximately one dozen professional newsletters (e.g., regional newsletters of the American Association on Mental Retardation; the newsletter of Division 33 of the American Psychological Association; the publication of the National Association of Private Residential Facilities for the Mentally Retarded, etc.) including a request that programs serving elderly mentally retarded individuals contact the project.

(5) Superintendents of the 282 public residential facilities for mentally retarded persons were contacted and asked to identify programs within their facilities for us to contact.

(6) The membership list of the National Association of Private Residential Facilities for the Mentally Retarded (NAPRFMR) was obtained. All member programs that did not have an upper age cutoff under 55 were contacted.

(7) A specialized list of programs responding to the 1982 census of community residential facilities conducted by the Center for Residential and Community Services of the University of Minnesota was provided to us. Residential programs in which at least 50% of the clients were aged 63 or older were identified by CRCS staff. (The structure of the census precluded generating a list of programs using age 55 as the cutoff point.) Programs on this list were then contacted by the project.

(8) Respondents from all programs included in the survey were asked to identify other potentially eligible programs for us to contact.

Each of these recruitment strategies yielded names of agencies, programs, and/or knowledgeable persons for us to contact. If a specific program's name was given, project staff conducted a screening telephone call to verify that the nominated program(s) met the study's inclusion criteria. If an agency name was given, the objective of the screening call was to identify all of the discrete programs sponsored by an agency that met study criteria. For example, if an agency provided a residential program composed of four group homes, each group home was screened to determine its eligibility. If an individual's name was provided to the project, the person was contacted to determine any programs or agencies known to him/her that should then be screened for inclusion in the study.

The task of identifying programs required the development of guidelines by which potentially eligible programs (e.g., a group home, a day habilitation program, a leisure skills development program) could be differentiated from the larger programmatic unit (e.g., the agency's residential component, a sheltered workshop, a community care center) within which the program was administratively lodged. In most instances, it was relatively easy to identify discrete programs within a service type. The following guidelines were effective in identifying the majority of the programs:

(1) The program had its own site or specified space within a larger site.
(2) The program had its own staff.
(3) The program had specific client entry criteria or was organized to serve specific types of clients.
(4) The program was offered at least three hours per week (this criterion pertained primarily to recreational or social activities programs).
(5) The program had its own budget (in community-based programs).

These guidelines were used as probes during the screening calls to identify discrete programs or to differentiate segments of larger programs. For example, if an agency operated a sheltered workshop that included several different components based on clients' functional or age characteristics, each component was screened as a separate program. These probes were useful in assisting the respondent to think about the sheltered workshop as a collection of discrete programs, any one of which might meet our study's criteria. Similarly, in screening institutionally based programs, a residential building that contained four wards or units was treated as, potentially, four programs if any of the first four guidelines described above were met. Each ward or unit was screened to determine its eligibility for the study.

These probes were also useful in distinguishing between individually based services and organized programs. For the purposes of this study, unique services (e.g., case advocacy, legal assistance) provided on an as-needed basis were not considered programs or included in the survey.

Table 3-1 presents the results of the program identification and screening processes for community-based programs described above. Of the 1,235 programs identified, 896 (72.5%) were screened out of the study. The most common reasons for excluding a program included: the program did not provide services to mentally retarded persons, the program had no specialized program for elders, or it did not meet our first inclusion criterion requiring that at least 50% of the mentally retarded persons served were age 55 or over. The relatively few programs ($n = 12$ or 3.5%) not included in the survey because of an

TABLE 3-1

Results of Program Identification and Screening Procedures:
Community-Based Programs

Number of programs identified	1,235	
Number of programs excluded	896	
Reasons for exclusion:		
(1) Did not serve MR persons or did not have special programs for elderly MR		376 (42.0%)
(2) Did not meet 50% rule		383 (42.7%)
(3) Did not meet 10% rule		30 (3.4%)
(4) Had only one MR person over age 55		44 (4.9%)
(5) Program opened after 1/1/85		12 (1.3%)
(6) Unable to contact		10 (1.1%)
(7) Other		41 (4.6%)
Number of eligible programs	339	
Number of refusals	12	
Number of programs surveyed	327	

unwillingness to participate is particularly impressive. As Table 3-1 indicates, 327 community-based programs were included in the survey.

Table 3-2 presents comparable information for institutionally based programs. As described earlier, the superintendents of 282 public residential facilities were contacted by the project and asked to identify programs that could potentially meet study criteria. Of the 282 institutions contacted, 62 (21.9%) did not respond to either our initial or followup inquiries. However, information regarding programs in six of these nonresponding institutions was offered by other sources and these institutional programs were subsequently included in the survey.

Of the 220 institutions that did respond, 158 (71.8%) had no programs that met the study's criteria. Thus, the 62 institutions included in the study represented 56 institutions responding to our requests for information and six institutions referred to the project by other sources as having potentially relevant programs. From these institutions, 202

TABLE 3-2

Results of Program Identification and Screening Procedures:
Institutionally Based Programs

Number of institutions contacted	282	
Number of institutions responding	220	(78.0%)
Number responding with no programs meeting study criteria	158	(71.8%)
Number of institutions with programs in the survey	62	
Number of institutionally based programs in the 62 institutions	202	

programs were identified as meeting the study's criteria and included in the survey.

PHASE III: DATA COLLECTION

The data were collected through telephone interviews conducted by trained research assistants. For each program, the appropriate respondent was contacted, given a detailed description of the interview process, and asked to schedule an appointment for the interview. The respondent was given the option of having one section of the interview sent to him/her in advance. This section contained questions requiring client-specific information that in larger programs would be difficult to assemble during the telephone interview. The information was then recorded by project staff during the scheduled interview.

The interview protocol consisted of a core set of questions asked of all programs and a separate set of questions depending on whether the program was residential or day program. Both structured and semistructured questions were used.

The core set of questions covered the following issues:

(1) history of the program;
(2) characteristics of currently served clients;
(3) program sponsorship;
(4) program funding;
(5) characteristics of the program's physical setting;
(6) types of service provided;
(7) special program issues in serving elderly mentally retarded persons.

Table 3-3 presents a detailed listing of the questions covered within each of these seven sections and within the residential and day sections of the protocol.

Two versions of the interview protocol were developed, one for community-based programs and one for institutionally based programs.* While both versions covered the above listed sections, different formats for some questions were needed to accommodate the different structural and administrative characteristics of institutions and community-based programs.

The respondents' positions within the agency or program are shown in Table 3-4. Administrators of community-based programs were the most common respondents, while program staff were the most common respondents for institutionally based programs.

---

* Copies of the interview protocols can be obtained from the authors.

TABLE 3-3

Description of Interview Content Areas

SECTION	TOPICS COVERED	NUMBER OF QUESTIONS COMMUNITY VERSION	NUMBER OF QUESTIONS INSTITUTIONAL VERSION
Core Questions			
1. History of the program	• when program began operation • when program began serving elderly MR • how decision was made to focus on this client group	6	5
2. Characteristics of currently served clients	• age • sex • level of mental retardation • other disabilities • health status	6	9
3. Program sponsorship	• status of program as private vs. public and for-profit vs. not-for-profit • other programs sponsored by the agency	3	NA
4. Program funding	• receipt of special grants • annual operating budget in 1984 • sources of funding in 1984	4	2
5. Physical setting	• type of neighborhood (urban, suburban, rural) • socioeconomic status of neighborhood • types of buildings located nearby • type of building • renovation status	3	3 2
6. Services	• which of 18 types of services are provided to elderly MR and younger MR clients • respondents' judgments of adequacy of services • transportation services • use of generic senior citizens programs and receptivity of such programs to elderly MR persons	7	8
7. Special program issues for elderly MR people	• which of six issues (e.g., death & dying, retirement) they have encountered and how they responded • respondents' judgments regarding special needs of elderly MR persons and how such special needs have shaped program characteristics • staff training on aging • program changes expected during the next two years • recommendations for other programs	7	11

TABLE 3-3

Description of Interview Content Areas (Continued)

SECTION	TOPICS COVERED	NUMBER OF QUESTIONS COMMUNITY VERSION	INSTITUTIONAL VERSION
Program Specific Questions			
8. Questions for residential programs only	• type of program (group home, foster home, etc.) • type of building • types and number of staff members • prior residences of current clients • vocational placements of current clients • retirement options • impact of having retired clients on program operation	6	12
9. Questions for nonresidential programs only	• type of program (day activity center, recreational program, etc.) • number of hours per week that clients attend • extent of physical and social integration of the elderly MR clients with other clients • types and numbers of staff members • residential placements of current clients	8	8

The interviews lasted an average of 70 minutes. The average length of time needed for community-based programs was 57.7 minutes, while for institutionally based programs the average was 81.7. Respondents for community-based programs were also asked to send us brochures, program descriptions, or other written materials about their programs and 38.5% did so.

A total of 529 programs were surveyed. Their distribution according

TABLE 3-4

Position of Respondent for Community- and Institution-Based Residential and Day Programs ($N = 529$)

	COMMUNITY-BASED RESIDENTIAL		DAY		INSTITUTION-BASED RESIDENTIAL		DAY	
POSITION OF RESPONDENT	n	%	n	%	n	%	n	%
Executive Director of sponsoring agency	23	12.0	23	17.0	n.a.		n.a.	
Administrator	90	46.9	62	46.0	51	35.4	27	46.6
Staff member	79	41.1	50	37.0	93	64.6	31	53.4
TOTAL	192	100%	135	100%	144	100%	58	100%

to location (institution or community-based) and type of service (residential or day) is shown in Table 3-5. The *National Directory of Programs Serving Elderly Mentally Retarded Persons* (Krauss, Seltzer, Howard, Litchfield, & Post, 1986) contains the names, addresses, and phone numbers of participating programs and institutions who agreed to be listed in the Directory.

LIMITATIONS OF THE SAMPLE

The strategies we used for assembling the pool of programs are subject to a number of limitations. Although our efforts to identify agencies, programs, and contact persons were both intensive and extensive, undoubtedly there were programs that met our study criteria but were missed. Thus, we did not study the full population of potentially eligible programs nor did we obtain a probability sample. Our sampling strategy was dependent upon the willingness of key informants, such as commissioners of state departments of mental retardation, to identify programs or agencies for us and upon the willingness of programs not known to such state agencies to contact us. We sent and received literally thousands of letters, but the number of programs that slipped through this net cannot be estimated.

There are, however, a number of factors that attest to the credibility of the sample we obtained. First, we received responses from at least one state agency official (usually the Commissioner of Mental Retardation) in each of the 50 states.

Second, we accessed multiple formal networks (e.g., the ARCs, NAPRFMR, regional and area office systems within the states) and informal networks (program known to other programs). There was only a modest degree of overlap in nominated programs across lists provided by formal and informal sources. Thus, a probability sample drawn from any one list would have underrepresented the true population of eligible programs.

TABLE 3-5

Distribution of Sample by Type of Setting and Type of Program ($N = 529$)

	TYPE OF SETTING		
TYPE OF PROGRAM	COMMUNITY-BASED	INSTITUTION-BASED	TOTAL
Residential	192	144	336
Day	135	58	193
TOTAL	327	202	529

Third, we received a very high rate of cooperation from programs potentially in our sample. Indeed, the enthusiasm and assistance we encountered in our hundreds of written and telephone inquiries was critical to our ability to track down many of the partial addresses or otherwise incomplete references we obtained. The large number of programs that responded but did not meet our criteria (see Table 3-1) and the very low rate of refusals from eligible programs (1%) attest to the generous spirit of the many administrators, program directors, and other program staff who gave graciously of their time and knowledge.

Specialized Programs Serving Elderly Mentally Retarded Persons

Chapter 4

National Distribution and Development
of Programs

This chapter presents information from the National Survey regarding four issues:

- The *national distribution* of programs serving elderly mentally retarded persons and the extent of state-to-state variability.
- The *history of programs* serving elderly mentally retarded persons, including year of opening and the extent to which they were created specifically to serve this population.
- The *organizational contexts* of such programs, including type of sponsoring agency, whether the agency sponsors other programs, and whether the other sponsored programs serve mentally retarded persons, nonretarded elderly, or other types of client groups.
- The *funding* of community-based programs serving elderly mentally retarded persons, including the 1984 per client costs, the sources of funds, and the use of special grants for program development.

The purpose of this chapter is therefore to describe the kinds of linkages these programs have to established service systems in the mental retardation and aging fields.

BACKGROUND

There is a great deal of variability among states in the number of programs for elderly mentally retarded persons that have been developed, in the extent to which this population has been targeted by state aging and developmental disabilities planning agencies, and in the availability of special state funding for programs serving this client group. This diversity exists in part because the development of programs for elderly mentally retarded persons began largely as a grassroots movement in response to needs identified by operators of programs for retarded adults approaching old age, by families of aging retarded persons, and by advocacy organizations. In some states, agencies such as the Department of Mental Retardation and the Department of Aging responded to the needs of this group after programs had already begun operation (Janicki, Ackerman, & Jacobson, 1985). In other states, no formal response (e.g., policy statements, guidelines, funding allocations) has yet been articulated.

The state-to-state diversity is also attributable to differences in the extent of interagency cooperation between the states' agencies responsible for persons with mental retardation and for aging or elderly persons. Janicki, Ackerman, and Jacobson (1985) found in their survey of mandated plans from the Developmental Disability Planning Councils (DDPC) and the state units on aging that about one-half of the DDPC's plans and only one-tenth of the state unit on aging's plans made specific reference to older persons with developmental disabilities. It was further reported that there was a very low rate of interagency agreement among agencies for mental retardation, aging, and/or the DDPCs regarding joint activities for this population. While a number of analysts have recommended more intensive collaboration among state agencies responsible for health care programs, services for the elderly, and services for the mentally retarded/developmentally disabled (Janicki, Knox, & Jacobson, 1985; Stone & Newcomer, 1985), contemporary practice suggests that state agencies for mental retardation/developmental disabilities will have to assume the lead agency role.

Only limited national data about the number of programs serving elderly mentally retarded persons were available at the time the National Survey was initiated. The 1982 National Census of Residential Facilities conducted by the Center for Residential and Community Services at the University of Minnesota identified licensed residential programs serving elderly mentally retarded persons (Hauber, Rotegard, & Bruininks, 1985). These data were limited, however, by three factors: only residential programs were surveyed; programs serving older mentally retarded persons between the ages of 55 and 63 and programs in which less than 100% of the clients were age 63 or older were not included in the analysis; and programs developed in response to the burgeoning but very recent interest in aging and retardation may not have been in operation in 1982. With these limitations in mind, they reported that in 1982 there were 293 residential facilities in the U.S. in which all of the mentally retarded persons surveyed were age 63 or older. While the average year of opening for these residences was 1974, half had opened between January 1, 1977, and June 30, 1982. The vast majority of these programs (89%) were sponsored by individuals, partners, or families; very few were operated by the formal service system. Thus, the recent (post-1982) response of the formal service system to the elderly mentally retarded population remains largely undocumented.

NATIONAL DISTRIBUTION OF PROGRAMS IN THE NATIONAL SURVEY

Table 4-1 shows the number of community and institutionally based residential and day programs in each of the fifty states and the District of

TABLE 4-1

Distribution of Programs in the National Survey by State (N = 529)

	COMMUNITY-BASED RESIDENTIAL	DAY	INSTITUTIONALLY BASED RESIDENTIAL	DAY	TOTAL
Alabama	6	1	3	3	13
Alaska					0
Arizona		1			1
Arkansas					0
California	10	13	7	1	31
Colorado	1			1	2
Connecticut	3	7	1		11
Delaware		1		1	2
Florida		6	4	1	11
Georgia			2	1	3
Hawaii	1	1			2
Idaho		6			6
Illinois	1	3	3		7
Indiana	1	1	2		4
Iowa	4	1			5
Kansas					0
Kentucky					0
Louisiana			3		3
Maine	1	1		1	3
Maryland	2	2			4
Massachusetts	19	8	13	14	54
Michigan	4	8	1	1	14
Minnesota	16	6	1	1	24
Mississippi		1	2		3
Missouri	8	2	1		11
Montana	4	2			6
Nebraska	5	2	2	2	11
Nevada					0
New Hampshire	2	3		1	6
New Jersey	5		26	5	36
New Mexico	1				1
New York	31	32	35	15	113
North Carolina			5		5
North Dakota	2	1			3
Ohio	10	8	4	2	24
Oklahoma					0
Oregon	2	2			4
Pennsylvania	19	8	3		30
Rhode Island	2	2	3	3	10
South Carolina	1		6	1	8
South Dakota		1	4	1	6
Tennessee	5		2	2	9
Texas	4		6		10
Utah					0
Vermont			2		2
Virginia	1				1
Washington	1	5			6
West Virginia	16				16
Wisconsin	3				3
Wyoming			3	1	4
District of Columbia	1				1
TOTAL	192 (36.3%)	135 (25.5%)	144 (27.2%)	58 (11.0%)	529 (100%)

Columbia that participated in the National Survey.* Community-based residential programs were located in 33 states and the District of Columbia, while community-based day programs were found in 28 states. Twenty-nine states had institutionally based programs meeting the study's criteria.

New York State had the largest number of programs (either institutional or community based) in the National Survey (113 programs), followed by Massachusetts (54 programs), California (31 programs), and Pennsylvania (30 programs). The average number of programs per state, counting only those states in which programs of that type were located, was 5.65 for residential programs and 4.82 for day programs. Thus, while the number of community-based programs for elderly mentally retarded persons is not large nationally, the programs tend to be clustered geographically, allowing for the possibility of some between-program networking and collaboration.

FACTORS ASSOCIATED WITH PROGRAM DEVELOPMENT

In order to identify potential explanations for the variability in states' development of programs for elderly mentally retarded persons, a series of secondary analyses was conducted using data available from Janicki, Knox, and Jacobson (1985), Janicki, Ackerman, and Jacobson (1984, 1985), the Center for Residential and Community Services at the University of Minnesota (Hauber, Bruininks, Hill, Lakin, Scheerenberger, & White, 1984) and the U.S. Bureau of the Census. The variables in these analyses were the states' demographic characteristics (percentage of the state's population age 55 and over, estimated number of developmentally disabled persons age 55 and over), extent of state activity related to older mentally retarded persons (inclusion of information or funding activity for this population by each state's Developmental Disabilities Council), and number of residential facilities for mentally retarded persons in the state.

Four sets of comparisons (using student's *t* test) were conducted regarding these variables. First, states with any community-based residential programs were compared with states without such programs. Next, states with any community-based day programs were compared with states without such program. Third, states with institutionally based residential programs were compared with states without such programs.

---

* The community-based programs include programs described in detail in Chapters 5, 6, and 8. The institutionally based programs include those described in detail in Chapter 7.

Fourth, states with institutionally based day programs were compared with states without such programs.

The purpose of these analyses was to determine whether patterns in the development of programs for elderly mentally retarded persons were related to the conditions existing in each state (e.g., the age structure of the population, the number of mentally retarded persons, the services for mentally retarded persons, and the available funding). The results are presented in Tables 4-2, 4-3, 4-4, and 4-5.

States that had *community-based residential programs* for elderly mentally retarded persons had a larger estimated developmentally disabled population over age 55 and a greater number of residential facilities for mentally retarded persons in the state, and were more likely to have community-based day programs for elderly mentally retarded persons than states that had no community-based residential programs (see Table 4-2).

States that had *community-based day programs* for elderly mentally retarded persons had a higher percentage of population age 55 or older and a greater number of residential facilities for mentally retarded adults

TABLE 4-2

Mean Differences Between States With and Without Community-Based Residential Programs

CHARACTERISTIC	STATE HAS RESIDENTIAL PROGRAMS ($n = 33$)	STATE DOES NOT HAVE RESIDENTIAL PROGRAMS ($n = 18$)	t
Percent of state population≥ 55 years[a]	21.27	19.78	1.39
Estimated number of developmentally disabled persons ≥ 55 years[b]	4,627	2,388	2.17*
Number of residential facilities for MR persons in the state[c]	410	117	2.51*
Developmental disabilities state plan includes information/issues on older population[d]	.57	.35	1.41
Developmental disabilities council funds special projects related to older population[d]	.20	.11	0.71
State has community-based day programs for elderly MR[e]	.70	.33	2.62**
State has institutionally based residential programs for elderly MR[e]	.55	.39	1.06
State has institutionally based day programs for elderly MR[e]	.45	.28	1.23

[a] Source: U.S. Bureau of the Census.   [b] Source: Janicki, Knox, & Jacobson (1985).   [c] Source: Hauber, Bruininks, Hill, Lakin, Scheerenberger, & White (1984).   [d] Source: Janicki, Ackerman, & Jacobson (1984, 1985). Code: 0 = no 1 = yes.   [e] Source: National Survey of Programs Serving Elderly Mentally Retarded Persons. Code: 0 = no 1 = yes.
* = $p<.05$.   ** = $p<.01$.

TABLE 4-3

Mean Differences Between States With and Without Community-Based
Day Programs

CHARACTERISTIC	STATE HAS DAY PROGRAMS (n = 29)	STATE DOES NOT HAVE DAY PROGRAMS (n = 22)	t
Percent of state population≥ 55 years[a]	21.83	19.30	2.97**
Estimated number of developmentally disabled persons ≥ 55 years[b]	4,605	2,825	1.68
Number of residential facilities for MR persons in the state[c]	443	126	2.43*
Developmental disabilities state plan includes information/issues on older population[d]	.62	.33	1.96*
Developmental disabilities council funds special projects related to older population[d]	.27	.05	2.20*
State has community-based residential programs for elderly MR[e]	.79	.45	2.62**
State has institutionally based residential programs for elderly MR[e]	.59	.36	1.58
State has institutionally based day programs for elderly MR[e]	.48	.27	1.53

[a] Source: U.S. Bureau of the Census.   [b] Source: Janicki, Knox, & Jacobson (1985).   [c] Source: Hauber, Bruininks, Hill, Lakin, Scheerenberger, & White (1984).   [d] Source: Janicki, Ackerman, & Jacobson (1984, 1985). Code: 0 = no 1 = yes.   [e] Source: National Survey of Programs Serving Elderly Mentally Retarded Persons. Code: 0 = no 1 = yes.
$* = p < .05.$ $** = p < .01.$

in the state, and were more likely to discuss aging as an issue in the state developmental disabilities plan, more likely to have the state developmental disabilities council fund special projects for older developmentally disabled clients, and more likely to have community-based residential programs for elderly mentally retarded persons than states that had no community-based day programs (see Table 4-3).

States that had *institutionally based residential programs* for elderly mentally retarded persons had a larger estimated developmentally disabled population over the age of 55 and a greater number of residential facilities for mentally retarded persons within the state and were more likely to have the state developmental disabilities council fund special projects for older developmentally disabled adults and more likely to have institutionally based day programs for elderly mentally retarded persons than states that had no institutionally based residential programs (see Table 4-4).

States that had *institutionally based day programs* for elderly mentally retarded persons had a greater number of residential facilities for mentally

TABLE 4-4

Mean Differences Between States With and Without Institutionally Based Residential Programs

CHARACTERISTIC	STATE HAS RESIDENTIAL PROGRAMS (n = 25)	STATE DOES NOT HAVE RESIDENTIAL PROGRAMS (n = 26)	t
Percent of state population≥ 55 years[a]	21.52	19.99	1.80
Estimated number of developmentally disabled persons ≥ 55 years[b]	6,036	1,722	4.25***
Number of residential facilities for MR persons in the state[c]	519	102	2.88**
Developmental disabilities state plan includes information/issues on older population[d]	.48	.50	−.15
Developmental disabilities council funds special projects related to older population[d]	.30	.04	2.46*
State has community-based residential programs for elderly MR[e]	.72	.58	1.06
State has community-based day programs for elderly MR[e]	.68	.46	1.58
State has institutionally based day programs for elderly MR[e]	.64	.15	4.02***

[a] Source: U.S. Bureau of the Census. [b] Source: Janicki, Knox, & Jacobson (1985). [c] Source: Hauber, Bruininks, Hill, Lakin, Scheerenberger, & White (1984). [d] Source: Janicki, Ackerman, & Jacobson (1984, 1985). Code 0 = no 1 = yes. [e] Source: National Survey of Programs Serving Elderly Mentally Retarded Persons. Code 0 = no 1 = yes.
 * = $p<.05$. ** = $p<.01$.*** = $p<.001$.

retarded persons within the state, and were more likely to have the state's developmental disabilities council fund special projects for older developmentally disabled adults, and more likely to have institutionally based residential programs for elderly mentally retarded adults than states that had no institutionally based day program (see Table 4-5).

These analyses suggest that the probability of a state having programs for elderly mentally retarded persons is in part a function of: the number of residential facilities for mentally retarded person in the state (this variable was significant in all four analyses); whether the state developmental disabilities council provided special funds for such services (this variable was significant in three of the four analyses); and the estimated size of the state's population of developmentally disabled persons over the age of 55 (this variable was significant in two of the four analyses). The size of the state's aging population, whether the state's developmental disabilities plan discusses aging, and the existence of other programs for elderly mentally retarded persons were less prominent factors.

TABLE 4-5

Mean Differences Between States With and Without Institutionally Based Day Programs

CHARACTERISTIC	STATE HAS DAY PROGRAMS (n = 20)	STATE DOES NOT HAVE DAY PROGRAMS (n = 31)	t
Percent of state population≥ 55 years[a]	21.41	20.31	1.24
Estimated number of developmentally disabled persons ≥ 55 years[b]	5,046	3,057	1.51
Number of residential facilities for MR persons in the state[c]	530	162	2.05*
Developmental disabilities state plan includes information/issues on older population[d]	.47	.50	−.17
Developmental disabilities council funds special projects related to older population[d]	.37	.04	2.79**
State has community-based residential programs for elderly MR[e]	.75	.58	1.23
State has community-based day programs for elderly MR[e]	.70	.48	1.53
State has institutionally based residential programs for elderly MR[e]	.80	.29	4.02***

[a] Source: U.S. Bureau of the Census.   [b] Source: Janicki, Knox, & Jacobson (1985).   [c] Source: Hauber, Bruininks, Hill, Lakin, Scheerenberger, & White (1984).   [d] Source: Janicki, Ackerman, & Jacobson (1984, 1985).   [e] Source: National Survey of Programs Serving Elderly Mentally Retarded Persons.
 * = $p<.05$.   ** = $p<.01$.   *** = $p<.001$.

HISTORY OF PROGRAMS

Programs serving elderly mentally retarded persons have developed either because existing programs have modified or internally restructured their services for this population (*evolved* programs) or because new programs were initiated with the express purpose of serving this population (*created* programs). Table 4-6 shows the number of programs in the National Survey that had evolved ($n = 256$ or 48.4%) or were created ($n = 273$ or 51.6%) to serve elderly mentally retarded persons. It also shows that about half of the community-based day ($n = 72$ or 53.3%) and residential ($n = 87$ or 45.3%) programs were intentionally created to serve older mentally retarded persons. Almost three-quarters of the institutionally based day programs ($n = 43$ or 74.1%) and about half of the institutionally based residential programs ($n = 71$ or 49.3%) were created for this population. Thus, in both institutional and community settings, day programs for elderly mentally retarded persons are more commonly

TABLE 4-6

Distribution of Programs as Evolved or Created to Serve Elderly Mentally Retarded Persons ($N = 529$)

| PROGRAM CHARACTERISTICS | COMMUNITY-BASED | | INSTITUTIONALLY-BASED | | |
| | RESIDENTIAL | DAY | RESIDENTIAL | DAY | |
	n	n	n	n	TOTAL
Evolved	105	63	73	15	256
Created	87	72	71	43	273
TOTAL	192	135	144	58	529

new programs designed for this target group while residential programs are often modifications of existing programs.

Obviously, our program identification procedures (see Chapter 3) were designed to locate such specially created programs. From this perspective, it is perhaps even more interesting that almost half of the community-based day and residential programs meeting the study's criteria were "evolved" programs (i.e., not originally designed to serve the aging population). These programs had either internally restructured their services or were simply serving a group of clients who had aged over time and now constituted a majority of the clients served.

Figure 4-1 illustrates when programs in the National Survey first served elderly mentally retarded persons. The recency and rate of growth of programs for elderly mentally retarded persons are striking. The peak year of program development for community-based residential and day programs was 1984. For institutionally based residential programs it was 1983, and for institutionally based day programs it was 1984. It is also notable that institutionally based day programs were the last to develop their first program (no programs prior to 1973), whereas each of the other types had at least one program in the 1960s. The factors accountable for the recent growth in the development of programs for this population warrant further investigation. What is notable, however, is that program initiation is a phenomenon of the early to mid-1980s.

Table 4-7 presents these data broken down by type of program and whether the program was created or evolved. As shown, created programs tend to be newer than evolved programs and day programs tend to be newer than residential programs. The oldest programs in the National Survey are the evolved institutionally based residential programs; the newest are the created community-based day programs. As will be shown in Chapters 5 through 7, although institutions were historically the first to respond to the needs of elderly mentally retarded persons, the community-based service system has become more active in recent years. Further, the recency of created community-based day

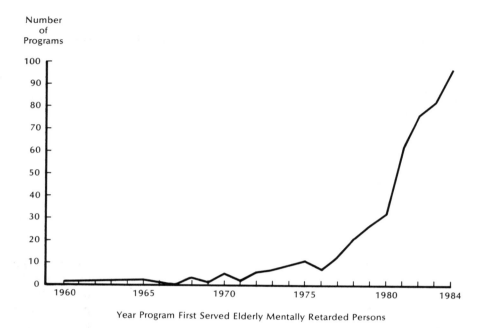

FIGURE 4-1:   Year for Institutionally and Community-Based Programs when Programs First Served Elderly Mentally Retarded Persons

programs may reflect the field's current focus on retirement options for elderly mentally retarded persons.

TABLE 4-7

Average Year Program Began Serving Elderly Mentally Retarded Persons

TYPE OF PROGRAM	EVOLVED	CREATED
Community-based residential	1978	1980
Community-based day	1980	1982
Institutionally based residential	1977	1980
Institutionally based day	1981	1981

ORGANIZATIONAL CONTEXT
OF COMMUNITY-BASED PROGRAMS

Table 4-8 presents information about the sponsoring agencies that operate community-based programs for elderly mentally retarded per-

TABLE 4-8

Types of Sponsoring Agencies of Community-Based Residential and Day Programs

SPONSORING AGENCIES	RESI-DENTIAL n	%	DAY n	%	χ^2
Type of Agency					
Public	27	14.1	41	30.4	
Private nonprofit	98	51.0	91	67.4	
Private for profit	39	20.3	3	2.2	
Individual operator	28	14.6	0	0.0	50.37***
Agency sponsors other programs for mentally retarded persons	129	82.7	120	91.6	4.17*
Agency sponsors other programs for non-mentally retarded elders	39	25.0	33	25.2	n.s.

$^* = p<.05.$ $^{***} = p<.001.$

sons. (As all institutionally based programs were sponsored by public residential facilities, these programs were omitted from this analysis.) As shown in Table 4-8, there was a significant difference between community-based residential and day programs ($\chi^2 = 50.37$, $p<.001$) with respect to their types of sponsoring agencies. About two-thirds of the day programs were sponsored by private non-profit agencies, compared with one-half of the residential programs. While 14.6% of the residential programs were sponsored by individual operators, none of the day programs lacked an organizational sponsor.

Virtually all (97%) of the community-based day programs were sponsored by multiprogram agencies, as compared with slightly over three-quarters (79%) of the residential programs ($\chi^2 = 20.39$, $p<.001$). The vast majority of the multiprogram agencies for both day and residential programs served mentally retarded persons in their other programs (91.6% and 82.7%, respectively), while about a fourth also served elderly clients who were not mentally retarded.

In summary, the program for elderly mentally retarded persons was rarely the only program operated by the sponsoring agency. Thus, the degree of structural integration within the traditional mental retardation and, to a lesser extent, aging service networks was high.

Informal contacts among community-based programs serving elderly mentally retarded persons were less common. Respondents from almost one-half of the evolved day programs knew of other specialized programs for this population. However, respondents from less than one-third of the created day programs, the created residential programs, and the evolved residential programs knew of even one other program.

The need for informal networking among programs serving this population is evident. When programs participating in the National Survey were asked whether they wished to be listed in the *National Directory of Programs Serving Elderly Mentally Retarded Persons* (Krauss, Seltzer, Howard, Litchfield, & Post, 1986), fully 92% of the community-based programs agreed to be listed.

FUNDING OF COMMUNITY-BASED PROGRAMS

Community-based programs were asked about their sources of funds in 1984 and the size of the 1984 budget. The average cost per client was derived by dividing the program's 1984 budget by the total number of clients served. As expected, there were significant differences in the average cost per client between the day (mean cost = $5,340.06) and residential (mean cost = $18,084.03) programs surveyed ($t = 4.72$, $p<.001$). There were also significant differences in the number of funding sources utilized by the two types of programs ($t = -5.44$, $p<.001$). Day programs averaged 2.15 sources of funds, compared with 2.93 sources for residential programs.

Table 4-9 provides information about the proportion of community-based programs that received funding in 1984 from each of 12 sources, broken down by evolved versus created and residential versus day. There was no significant difference in the funding patterns for evolved as compared with created programs. In contrast, residential and day programs received funds from different sources, with residential programs more likely to receive client fees (SSI, Social Security, SSDI,

TABLE 4-9

Funding Sources for Community-Based Programs ($N = 327$)

FUNDING SOURCES	EVOLVED n	CREATED n	χ^2	RESIDENTIAL n	DAY n	χ^2
Title XX	14	8	2.72	5	19	14.06***
State program funds	91	100	2.05	134	96	0.12
Vocational rehab. funds	0	2	0.31	0	3	2.25
Medicaid	41	66	2.44	76	51	0.01
Medicare	12	9	0.95	13	12	0.29
SSI	55	54	2.15	125	11	101.97***
SS retirement	36	33	1.76	77	6	50.49***
SSDI	13	12	0.32	27	4	9.88***
Private client fees	14	27	1.67	40	15	4.45*
Special federal grants	0	2	0.31	2	1	0.07
Special state grants	3	3	0.00	1	6	4.19*
Special private grants	14	8	2.72	12	15	1.99

$* = p<.05.$ $*** = p<.001.$

private fees) and day programs more likely to receive Title XX funds and special state grants.

Respondents were asked if special funds had been received to initiate their programs for older mentally retarded persons. About one-quarter of the community-based day programs (26.9%) had received special grants during the first year of operation for this population, compared with about a fifth of the community-based residential programs (21.5%). Respondents from about one-third (36.8%) of the day programs and one-quarter (25.1%) of the residential programs reported that the program had subsequently received special funds for their activities. Interestingly, no significant differences were found between evolved and created programs in the receipt of special funds, either during the first year of operation or subsequently.

CONCLUSIONS

This chapter presented information on the distribution and organizational characteristics of the 327 community-based and 202 institutionally based programs serving elderly mentally retarded persons that were included in the National Survey. All but seven states had at least one program for this population. One state (New York) had over one hundred programs. Thus, there was evidence of programmatic development across the country although the highest concentrations of such activity were located in a very few states.

Some factors potentially contributing to state variability in specialized program growth were described. Our analyses suggest that growth is a function of need (the number of developmentally disabled persons over age 55 in the state), the existing strength of the community-based residential system (defined solely in terms of quantity), and policymaker awareness (defined in terms of recognition of this population in official planning documents).

1984 seems to have been the pivotal year in the development of both community- and institutionally based day programs and of community-based residential programs. The growth spurt illustrated in Figure 4-1 during the mid-1980s suggests that a confluence of factors—possibly need, strength of the residential systems, and professional and service provider awareness—resulted in the beginning of a very active period of development.

In this regard, it is particularly noteworthy that about half of the programs in the National Survey were modifications of existing programs and half were newly created to serve the elderly mentally retarded population. Obviously, an important issue for program planners and administrators is the elasticity of current program structures (Janicki,

Krauss, & Seltzer, in press). The results of the National Survey suggest that at least some of the current program structures are sufficiently flexible to enable these programs to serve different populations than originally intended. As will be discussed in Chapters 5 through 8, there is a great deal of diversity in residential and day program models for this population. Some of the models represent significant departures from or innovations in existing programs in the mental retardation services system. However, others bear a strong resemblance to traditional programs for mentally retarded persons.

Program growth for elderly mentally retarded persons seems to be located within established agencies providing multiple programs to mentally retarded and/or non-mentally retarded elders. This is another positive sign of the capacity of the existing service system to respond to new needs within the field. Further, there was an impressive diversity of funding sources used to support these programs. While the availability of special grants for program development is an obvious incentive, the majority of community-based programs were started and have been sustained without such funds.

In sum, there is reason for optimism in the continued growth of programs serving elderly mentally retarded persons. First, it is a national phenomenon. Second, programs are developing currently (mid-1980s) at a more rapid rate than ever before reported. Third, this growth is occurring primarily within the existing services structure and with the support of traditional sources of funds. These characteristics attest to the capacity for responsiveness to new needs that has long been a goal of advocates, service providers, and planners in the mental retardation field.

Chapter 5

Community-Based
Residential
_____Programs

This chapter presents descriptive information and analyses of the community-based residential programs that participated in the National Survey. It begins with a discussion of existing typologies of residential services for both the mentally retarded and elderly populations. A detailed discussion of the six-model classification scheme developed from the National Survey is then presented, followed by a comparative analysis of significant programmatic differences among the six models.

BACKGROUND

A variety of classification schemes of community-based residential programs have been proposed since the inception of the community residence movement. Classification schemes are useful for both descriptive and analytic purposes. Given the extent of interstate variability in the types and names for community residential programs (Hill & Lakin, 1986), the need for a common language to distinguish among program types remains a problem in research and policy analysis (Landesman-Dwyer, 1985). To date, no consensus has emerged regarding the most salient dimensions along which to classify program models (Campbell & Bailey, 1984). Existing typologies vary in their emphasis on such characteristics as licensure, size and function of the program, characteristics of the population served, and habilitation orientation.

Table 5-1 illustrates the variety of residential typologies proposed over the last ten years. They vary in terms of the number of classifications presented from a minimum of three (Butler & Bjaanes, 1977) to a maximum of 17 (Scheerenberger, 1983). They also vary with respect to their emphasis. Some (e.g., Scheerenberger, 1983) are essentially categorical listings of an array of services, while others (e.g., Butler & Bjaanes, 1977; Campbell & Bailey, 1984) classify programs by dimensions such as program philosophy or orientation. To some extent, these differences reflect the multiple purposes of classification schemes both as tools for comparative descriptions and as tools for analyzing the influence of different types of environments on client outcomes.

For example, Baker, Seltzer, and Seltzer's (1977) typology consisted of

TABLE 5-1

Residential Typologies

AUTHOR	TYPOLOGY	DIMENSIONS USED FOR CLASSIFICATION
Baker, Seltzer, & Seltzer (1977)	1. Small group homes (10 or fewer residents) 2. Medium group homes (11–20 residents) 3. Large group homes (21–40 residents) 4. Mini-institutions (41–80 residents) 5. Mixed group homes 6. Group homes for older adults 7. Foster family care 8. Sheltered villages 9. Workshop dormitories 10. Community preparatory programs 11. Semi-independent units 12. Comprehensive systems	● Type of administrative structure ● Characteristics of served population ● Program philosophy ● Size of program
Butler & Bjaanes (1977)	1. Custodial 2. Maintaining 3. Therapeutic	● Presence of habilitative programming ● Degree of community contact ● Level of activity within the residence ● Intensity of caregiver involvement
Campbell & Bailey (1984)	Family Oriented 1. Natural family 2. Foster family 3. Boarding home Client directed 4. Independent living Agency directed 5. Group home	
Hill & Lakin (1986)	1. Specialized foster home 2. Small group residence (1–6/7–15) 3. Large private group residence (16–63/64–299/300+) 4. Large public group residence (16–63/64–299/300+) 5. Semi-independent 6. Board and supervision 7. Personal care 8. Specialized nursing	● Program model ● Size of program

TABLE 5-1
Residential Typologies (Continued)

AUTHOR	TYPOLOGY
Scheerenberger (1983)	1. Natural family home 2. Foster family home 3. Group home 4. Private residential facility 5. Semi-independent living 6. Independent living 7. Boarding home 8. Community psychiatric program 9. General medical hospital 10. Public residential facility 11. Hospital for the mentally ill 12. Nursing home 13. Correctional facility 14. School for the blind 15. Intermediate care facility 16. Rest home 17. Work placement

12 types defined according to administrative structure, characteristics of the population served, program philosophy, and size of the program. Butler and Bjaanes' (1977) three-model typology used the following dimensions for classification purposes: presence of habilitative programming, degree of community contact, level of activity within the residence, and intensity of caregiver involvement. Campbell and Bailey's (1984) typology reflected the sponsorship of the program. More recently, Hill and Lakin (1986) presented a typology based on three variables: program model, size, and sponsorship.

Just as mental retardation researchers and planners have attempted to classify residential services provided to mentally retarded persons, so too have gerontologists developed typologies with respect to residential services for elderly persons. It is commonly noted that the vast majority of older persons in this country live in "unplanned" housing, most commonly in their own homes or with relatives (Huttman, 1985). For the 8% who live in planned or specially designed housing environments for senior citizens, a number of types exist. Huttman (1985) describes three general types of programs for seniors: apartment complexes, congregate housing, and retirement communities. Apartment complexes include public housing projects and nonprofit and privately owned housing complexes. In these settings, residents typically do their own cooking and housekeeping with varying levels of ancillary services provided by the housing authorities.

Congregate housing differs from apartment complexes primarily in the range and intensity of services provided. Meals, heavy housekeeping, and other personal and recreational services are usually provided by staff. Limited health services and an infirmary are often available. Residents usually do not have their own kitchen facilities and may live in hotel-type rooms. Also included in the congregate housing type are *life care communities* (Pies, 1984) or, as they have more recently been termed, *continuing care communities* (Branch, 1987). In such facilities, a resident buys the apartment or townhouse in which they live. If nursing care is needed, it is provided on site as part of the community's services. The life care community guarantees lifelong care to the resident commensurate with his/her level of need. Life care communities provide a broad array of services, including meals, housekeeping, recreational programs, and comprehensive medical care.

Retirement villages or communities are age-segregated, noninstitutional communities often located in the sun belt, retirement areas, or peripheries of urban areas. Residents often purchase their living units. As in life care communities, retirement communities frequently cater to the middle class and affluent economic group of elderly and may support both retail and service economies separate from the larger community in which they are located. A variety of services are often available in such programs, with particular emphasis on recreational activities.

A more detailed typology of age-segregated residential settings for older persons was presented by Gelwicks (1984). This typology categorizes housing into five groups, ranging from housing for highly independent individuals to the controlled environment of the nursing home. The first type includes settings in which services are provided on a fee-for-service basis and initiated by the individual. These settings include retirement community detached homes, housing for the elderly, mobile home parks, retirement hotels, and shared housing. The second type includes settings in which at least one meal is provided for residents and in which managers assume some responsibility for the well-being of the residents. These settings include congregate housing, a child's or relative's home, and retirement living centers. The third type includes relatively small settings in which residents receive some assistance in daily living tasks but not skilled nursing care. Examples of residences in the group are board and care homes and residential care or assisted care living facilities. The fourth group includes residences in which a wide range of services and facilities (including health care) are available for both independent and dependent elderly persons. Settings such as homes for the aging, continuing care retirement communities, or life care communities are examples of this type. The final group consists of settings that provide complete care for totally dependent individuals, such as nursing homes, intermediate care facilities, skilled nursing facilities, and geriatric hospitals.

To date, no residential typology has been offered specifically for programs serving elderly mentally retarded persons. There are, however, studies that describe the residential placements of various age cohorts of mentally retarded persons. The Center for Residential and Community Services at the University of Minnesota conducted a national census of residential facilities for persons with mental retardation in 1982. From their national sample of 15,633 facilities, they extracted information on 603 residents who lived in settings in which all of the clients served were age 63 and over (see Hauber, Rotegard, & Bruininks, 1985, for a complete discussion of the findings). Over half (55.7%) of the 603 residents were living in foster homes, 15.5% lived in group homes serving 15 or fewer residents, 13.6% lived in personal care homes, 7.6% were in nursing homes, 4.6% were in large group homes (16 to 63 residents), 2.8% were in boarding homes, and the remaining 0.2% were in supervised apartments.

Data from the 1977 National Nursing Home Survey indicate that approximately 42,000 persons whose primary diagnosis is mental retardation lived in nursing homes (Lakin, 1985). Over half of these residents were age 55 or older.

Other studies have described the residential placement patterns within specific states. For example, Janicki and MacEachron (1984) reported the residential placements as of 1982 for three age cohorts of mentally retarded persons in New York State: late middle age (ages 53–62), aging (ages 63–72), and aged (ages 73–99). Their survey included all persons over the age of 53 living in developmental centers and community-based residential programs in New York State. The results indicated that with advancing age, there were increases in the percentage of persons living in developmental centers and/or congregate care centers (50%, 54%, and 62%, respectively for the three age cohorts), foster homes (18%, 23%, and 25%, respectively), and adult board and care homes (2%, 5%, and 6%, respectively). Conversely, the percentage of persons living in community residences decreased with advancing age (14%, 9%, and 4%, respectively) as did the percentage of persons living either alone or with relatives (15%, 8%, and 2%, respectively).

Rowitz (1980) found that the residential placements of 232 persons aged 50 and over served by a regional center in California were as follows: 30.3% in family foster care, 24.1% in group homes, 15.9% in nursing homes, 11.2% with their parents, 9.1% in public institutions, 4.7% in independent living situations, and the remaining 5.0% were living in other settings.

In a more recent study of the residential placements of 59,000 mentally retarded persons in California, Meyers, Borthwick, and Eyman (1985) reported that over half (52.5%) lived in their natural family homes. This proportion varied with ethnicity, severity of retardation, and age of the person. However, at age 55, about a quarter of all mildly retarded persons, a fifth of moderately retarded persons, 8% of severely retarded persons, and about 3% of profoundly retarded persons were still living with their natural families.

Finally, Krauss and Seltzer (1984) reported that mentally retarded persons aged 55 to 74 who were receiving state supported services in Massachusetts were living in a variety of settings. Almost three-quarters (74.2%) lived in state schools or institutions, 13.9% lived in community residences, 10.1% lived in a nursing home, and the remaining 1.8% lived with family members.

While these state and national studies vary in scope, definitions of residential settings, and period of data collection, it is possible to extract common findings from them. First, a majority of the mentally retarded elderly population lives in institutional or congregate care settings and the percentage of this population so placed increases with age. Second, foster homes (sometimes called *family foster care* or *specialized family care*) are a frequently used community-based residential placement for this age group (see also Seltzer et al., 1982; Sherman, et al., 1984). Third, while group homes are also commonly used, the percentage of elderly mentally retarded persons living in such settings decreases with advancing age.

Clearly, then, existing residential typologies as illustrated in Table 5-1 include the types of programs in which older mentally retarded persons live. For this population, no distinctive type of residential program has been described that departs from the widely used categories of group homes, foster homes, board and care homes and public institutions.

THE RESIDENTIAL TYPOLOGY

There were 186 community-based residential programs included in the National Survey. (In Chapter 4, the number of community-based programs was given as 192. Six of these programs, located in large privately operated residential facilities, are analyzed separately in Chapter 8.) These 186 programs were subjected to a qualitative case-by-case review. This process generated the identification of six types, which were then used as the independent variables in the quantitative analyses described in the sections that follow. Table 5-2 presents the distribution of these programs across the six categories. Qualitative and quantitative information is presented on each of the models below. A comparative analysis among the residential models is then presented.

TABLE 5-2

Typology of Community-Based Residential Programs

TYPE	N	%
Foster homes	26	14.0
Group homes	50	26.9
Group homes with nurses	27	14.5
Intermediate care facilities for the mentally retarded	44	23.7
Apartment programs	19	10.2
Mixed residential programs	20	10.7
TOTAL	186	100.0

Foster Homes

Foster homes are licensed residences in which a pre-existing household accepts nonfamily members into the home. These providers are usually required to have some specialized training or experience, but the homes vary in the extent to which habilitative services are provided as part of the service agreement. Twenty-six foster homes were included in the National Survey.

This category includes residences that were self-described by respondents by many names, including foster homes and board and care or boarding homes. Our criteria for inclusion in this model were that the residence be small in size (less than four residents) and individually operated (although some foster homes were affiliated with a foster care agency).

The foster homes were located in ten different states, with the largest number (nine of the 26 homes) in West Virginia alone. In general, foster homes in the National Survey were homes in which long term residents had simply aged into the 55 and over category. Most were initially opened to serve younger adults. For example, one home had served four women for over forty years. The average year in which the sampled foster homes began serving their residents was 1977, placing them among the oldest program types in the National Survey. This type of program was the second least expensive of the residential types, with an average cost per resident in 1984 of $5,474. None had ever received a special grant for providing services to elderly mentally retarded persons.

There were, on average, 5.50 residents for each staff person per home. This was the highest resident:staff ratio among any of the residential types. While about two-thirds of the foster homes had administrators and/or direct care staff, few employed any professional staff (i.e., occupational therapists, social workers, etc.). In spite of the nonprofessional composition of the staff, almost two-thirds (62%) of the foster home operators reported obtaining specialized training in the care of older mentally retarded persons for their staff.

Consistent with their low per-resident cost, foster homes provided the fewest number of services for their elderly mentally retarded residents of any of the community residential program types (an average of 4.9 services). The most commonly provided services were recreational/social activities, transportation, and assistance with self care. Few provided therapeutic or habilitative programming for the residents.

Foster homes, by definition small in size, served an average of 3.7 persons; most (3.2) of these persons were mentally retarded and over the age of 55. A third (33%) of the elderly mentally retarded persons in foster homes were described as mildly retarded, almost half (47%) as moderately retarded, and a fifth (20%) as severely or profoundly retarded. Almost two-thirds (64%) were female.

The average age of the residents in foster homes was 65.9 years. Most such homes (85%) served only persons over the age of 55. The health status of elderly mentally retarded residents, rated by respondents with respect to the residents' age and level of disability, was described as follows: 26% were in excellent health, 44% were in good health, 25% were in fair health, and 5% were in poor health.

Almost half (48%) of the elderly mentally retarded residents in foster homes had no formal day programs and thus spent their days at home with their foster families. In this respect, foster home residents were the second most "retired" group of residents (second only to the mixed residential programs described below). Almost a fifth (17%) attended day activity centers while another 14% attended senior citizens' programs. Very few attended specialized day programs for elderly mentally retarded persons or vocationally oriented programs, or had formal programming at their residences.

In sum, foster homes in the National Survey (as is true for foster homes in general) can be characterized as a nonprofessional residential model. These programs had the fewest staff, provided the fewest services, and consequently constituted the second least expensive program model of any in the community residential typology. The providers of foster care were often responsible for their residents 24 hours per day because the majority of the residents had no day program. The amount of personal care provided in these homes was considerable, especially in light of the fact that a fifth of the elderly mentally retarded persons served were severely or profoundly retarded.

Group Homes

Group homes are professionally staffed residences for unrelated handicapped persons that provide residents with training in daily living activities, opportunities for recreation, and a supportive environment for the development of skills for increased independence. Although they vary greatly in size, the majority accommodate 15 or fewer residents (Hill & Lakin, 1986).

Fifty group homes were included in the National Survey, making this category the most common among the residential types. These homes were located in 18 states. Most (60%) were sponsored by private nonprofit agencies. Many of the sponsoring agencies provided a variety of programs to mentally retarded persons of all ages. For such agencies, the development of group homes for older clients completed their continuum of residential alternatives.

The average year in which these group homes served their first elderly mentally retarded person was 1981. Only one-third were specifically created to serve this population. Rather, most programmatically modified existing homes to meet the needs of aging residents.

Group homes averaged 6.9 clients, of whom 5.4 were over the age of 55. The average per client budget in 1984 was $15,240, comparable to apartment programs (discussed below). A third of the programs had received special grants for development of their programs for elderly mentally retarded persons, either during their first year of operation or subsequently.

There were on the average 1.8 residents per full-time staff person in these programs. Nearly all programs employed administrators (98%) and direct care staff (98%). About one-quarter had staff social workers and 16% employed teachers. Over half of the programs had provided specialized training to their staff in various aspects of aging and mental retardation.

These programs tended to offer the same array of training and community living experiences for their aging residents as is typically true for group homes serving younger adults. However, they perceived their program philosophy to be less goal oriented than did other group homes. For example, one respondent stated that the residents shouldn't "be programmed to death." The emphasis was more commonly placed on encouraging residents to make their own choices, to facilitate a more relaxed pace of activities, to access community-based resources for recreational and leisure activities, and to monitor nutritional needs and physical fatigue. While two-thirds of the programs had accessed community-based senior citizen services for at least one of their residents (the second highest among the residential types), staff frequently commented on the limited availability of programs or services for older mentally retarded persons. "There's just a lack of awareness that these people exist."

The residents in group homes averaged 61.85 years and the majority (53%) were female. There was considerable variability in the level of retardation of the elderly mentally retarded clients served. Forty percent were mildly retarded, 37% were moderately retarded and 23% were severely or profoundly retarded. While the majority were described as in either excellent or good health, a quarter (25%) were in either fair or poor health. The heterogeneity of the population with respect to level of retardation and health status has obvious programmatic implications. As one staff member cautioned, "With elderly clients, it is a mistake to mix many levels of functioning, because higher functioning clients don't get as much attention when the lower functioning clients require so much."

Staff in group homes saw a greater difference in the needs of their older residents as compared with their younger residents than in any of the other residential types. The most commonly expressed differences were that elderly mentally retarded persons had more specialized health care needs, lower energy and motivation levels, different friendship needs, and different activity preferences than did younger mentally retarded adults.

Most residents in these group homes went either to vocational programs (28%) or activity programs (21%) during the day. Almost one-fifth (18%) went to special day programs for elderly mentally retarded persons and 10% attended generic senior citizens' programs. Five percent were described as not involved in day programs, another 8% spent their days at the residence in formal programs, and 10% attended other types of day programs.

One of the most persistent issues described by staff in group homes was the need for relaxation in the day program schedules and/or retirement options for their residents. Thus, while most residents of these homes had day programs, there was considerable frustration expressed about their appropriateness. As one respondent put it, "the elderly are ignored in the day programs. Their emphasis is on *working* and the elderly have a right to retire."

In sum, group homes were the most prevalent community-based residential type in the National Survey. While their structural characteristics (number of clients, average costs, staffing patterns) mirror those of other group homes, these homes had modified their programmatic orientations in ways intended to enrich their residents' elder years. The emphasis was less on achieving new skills than on maintaining existing skills, less on staff-directed activities than on resident-initiated activities, less on exposing residents to new challenges than on supporting their need for a more relaxed pace.

Group Homes with Nurses

This category is similar to the group home category described above but with one important distinction. Twenty-seven group homes in the

National Survey each had a nurse on the staff. Because this represents an important staffing distinction, we differentiate between these two types of group homes.

The 27 group homes with nurses were located in 12 states, with ten in New York State alone. Most (52%) were sponsored by private nonprofit agencies, with an additional one-third (33%) sponsored by private for-profit agencies. Almost all were multiprogram agencies that sponsored other programs for mentally retarded and nonretarded elders.

Group homes with nurses served their first elderly mentally retarded person, on average, in 1980. Less than half (41%) were specifically created to serve this population. One program described its reason to start as resulting from its referrals, which were "skewed to the older population. We didn't really start out to have this type of program. It just sort of happened."

These group homes were the third largest in size of all the residential types and were slightly larger than group homes without nurses. The average size was 8.9 residents, of whom 6.3 were over the age of 55. The annual per client budget for 1984 was $22,089, the second highest of the residential types.

These homes averaged 1.3 residents per staff person. Group homes with nurses were slightly more professionally staffed residences than the group homes described above. In addition to administrators, direct care staff, and nurses, almost half employed social workers, a third employed psychologists, and a few employed physicians, teachers, and homemakers. The presence of a nurse as a regular member of the core staff signified an important modification of the group home model for serving older residents. Yet there was considerable variability in the manner in which the nurse was utilized. For example, in one residence the nurse spent one evening per month in the program, with additional visits as needed. In another, there was a full-time licensed practical nurse on the staff.

Group homes with nurses were a "service rich" program model, second only to the Intermediate Care Facilities for the Mentally Retarded (ICFs/MR, discussed below) in the average number of services provided. The majority provided a range of health, therapeutic, support, and social services to their residents.

Philosophically, these programs had similar goals to those described for group homes above. However, many had physically redesigned the program environment to accommodate the declining health of their residents. For example, one program recommended that single story dwellings be used to reduce the ambulation requirements of multiple story dwellings. Other programs stressed the rapidity with which physical, emotional, and biological effects of aging can occur and noted that residential programs must be attuned to these changes. It was encouraging to find that group homes with nurses were often strong advocates of physically modifying the home to accommodate resident needs rather than seeking a nursing home placement for residents whose physical capacities were diminishing. Thus, the programmatic emphasis was commonly placed on meeting the health care needs of clients, modifying the physical design and daily routine to reflect resident needs, and maintaining strong links with the medical community. These programs often characterized themselves as homelike alternatives to nursing home placement. One program noted that it had explored the option of being licensed as an intermediate care facility but decided that it would rather "stay as we are. We're more homelike."

Staff saw many differences in the needs of older as compared with younger mentally retarded clients. For example, one program was started in recognition that some older mentally retarded persons are not able or willing to continue to go to outside day programs. The respondent described the residence as a "retirement-like program that can meet residents' needs as senior citizens . . . in a semi-formal program of activities. The program targets those for whom the long term goal of semi-independent living or sheltered employment is no longer considered realistic."

While a third (32%) of the elderly mentally retarded residents were mildly retarded, 43% were moderately retarded, and 25% were severely or profoundly retarded. The majority (55%) of elderly mentally retarded residents in group homes with nurses were male. Despite emphasis on the needs of the aging population, these group homes had the youngest average age per client, 58.7 years. Further, the health status of the residents was not significantly worse than in any of the other residential models. Over a quarter (26%) of the residents were said to be in excellent health, 45% were rated as in good health, 23% in fair health, and 6% in poor health.

A third of the residents (33%) attended vocational programs during the day, while a fifth (19%) participated in day activity programs. Fourteen percent went to special day programs for elderly mentally retarded clients, while very few (1%) attended generic senior citizen programs. Other clients (14%) remained at the residence but participated in formal programs, while 12% remained at the residence with no formal program participation. The remaining clients (7%) attended other types of day programs. Many of the homes whose residents attended outside day programs noted the need to develop in-residence day programs and/or to access senior citizen programs more broadly.

In summary, group homes with nurses represented the most distinctive modification of an existing residential type found in the National Survey. These homes were characterized by their attention to the medical and health care needs of the residents while maintaining as typical a group home as possible. They clearly represent an important variant of the group home model with special significance to the growing number of elderly mentally retarded persons.

Intermediate Care Facilities for the Mentally Retarded (ICFs/MR)

Since 1971, Title XIX of the Social Security Act has authorized Medicaid funding for "care for the mentally retarded in public institutions which have the primary purpose of providing health and rehabilitation services and which are classified as intermediate care facilities." ICFs/MR are specially designated facilities that "furnish (in single or multiple facilities) food and shelter to four or more persons unrelated to the proprietor, and in addition, provide some treatment or services which meet some need beyond the basic provision of food and shelter" (Boggs, Lakin, & Clauser, 1985, pp. 1–57). In general, these programs are characterized by stringent staffing and treatment requirements, which exceed those typically found for other types of residential programs serving mentally retarded persons (Lakin, Hill, & Bruininks, 1985; Manfredini & Smith, in press).

Forty-four community-based ICFs/MR were identified in the National Survey. Sixteen were located in New York and 13 were in Minnesota. These two states are among the most active in the use of ICF/MR programs for serving mentally retarded persons of all ages (Lakin et al., 1985).

The average year in which these programs first served elderly mentally retarded persons was 1981, making this type of program, along with group homes, the second most recently developed of the residential types. Consistent with the recency of their providing services to elderly mentally retarded persons, almost three-quarters (71%) of these programs were specifically created to serve this older population, the highest percentage in the study. These programs were also the most expensive residential type, averaging $30,773 per client in 1984. Over half (55%) were sponsored by private nonprofit agencies, while a third (32%) were sponsored by private for-profit agencies.

There were on average 1.32 residents for each staff person. In addition to administrators, direct care staff, and nurses (employed by nearly all ICFs/MR), 66% employed social workers, 48% employed psychologists, and 43% had therapists as part of the staff. A quarter of these programs also employed physicians and/or homemakers. Almost all ICFs/MR (88%) indicated that staff had received specialized training in the needs of older mentally retarded persons, the highest percentage for any residential model.

ICFs/MR provided the highest average number of services to residents

(15.8 per program). For example, one program identified the following range of services: meal preparation, medication administration, nursing services, laundry and housekeeping services, resident funds management, transportation, social and recreational activities, and facility vacations. Further, this program also provided training in social development, household management, academic skills, home and community activities, and vocational preparation.

Most programs emphasized that residents need a slower pace of activities and that, as a result, programs were "less goal-oriented and more oriented towards leisure activities." However, programs were also characterized by their links to the medical and health care communities. Most programs noted that knowing about the medical aspects of aging and developing appropriate resources to care for deteriorating residents were primary goals of their programs.

ICFs/MR served an average of 17.0 residents per facility, of whom 13.4 were elderly mentally retarded persons. The average age of the residents was 62.6 years. Fully 42% of the elderly mentally retarded residents were severely or profoundly retarded. No other residential type served such a high percentage of comparably intellectually impaired persons. Interestingly, the health ratings for these residents were similar to those for other residential types'. Over three-quarters (75%) were reported to be in good or excellent health. One-fifth (21%) were judged to be in fair health, and only 4% were judged to be in poor health.

Almost a third (30%) of the elderly mentally retarded residents of ICFs/MR attended formal day programs at the facility, a considerably higher percentage than for any other residential program type. One-quarter (24%) attended sheltered workshops or vocationally oriented programs. Fifteen percent went to special day programs for elderly mentally retarded persons. Eight percent attended day activity programs. A relatively small percentage went to senior citizen programs (5%) or were at the residence with no formal programming (7%).

In sum, ICF/MR programs in the National Survey had the second highest average number of residents and provided the largest number of services. They were also the most expensive of the models. These programs had a large number of regulatory constraints by virtue of federally imposed mandates. However, many described themselves as capable of meeting the needs of older residents because of their diverse mixture of staff and services. While the required availability of medical and nursing staff enabled these programs to accept persons whose health status was expected to decline and for whom continued participation in outside day programs was not required, the current health of residents was no worse than in other residential models; it was in their cognitive abilities that residents of ICFs/MR were most impaired. Finally, these programs were more likely to provide formal day programming as part of the residential services than as any other residential model. In this respect, ICFs/MR were the most comprehensive "retirement" programs identified in the residential typology.

Apartment Programs

Apartment programs (sometimes called *semi-independent living programs*) are usually located in apartment buildings. One or more units are occupied by a group of mentally retarded individuals. Staff provide less than 24-hour-a-day supervision and may either live in the apartment complex or make visits on a routine basis. Residents are typically responsible for their own housekeeping, meal preparation, and basic living skills, although the degree of staff assistance provided varies (Halpern, Close, & Nelson, 1986).

Of the 19 apartment programs included in the National Survey, eight were in Massachusetts. Virtually all (90%) were sponsored by private, nonprofit, multiprogram agencies. Only a third (37%) were initially created to serve this older population.

The average year in which these programs served their first elderly mentally retarded resident was 1982. There were on average 1.6 residents per staff person. Apartment programs were not, however, frequent employers of professional staff. About a fifth (21%) of the programs had a teacher, while 16% had a social worker on staff. Thus, the bulk of the supervision and services provided in these programs were the responsibility of administrators and nonprofessional direct care staff. The average per client cost in 1984 of the apartment programs was $15,619, the third highest among the residential types.

Virtually all of the programs said there were differences in the needs of their older as compared with their younger mentally retarded residents. Specifically, many noted that environmental adaptations were needed in the apartments, that residents' medical needs differed, and that an increase in the number of staff was needed to adequately serve these older residents. One respondent noted that, "the elderly have trouble coping with increased dependence." Another noted that "the program must be flexible and have a good pacing to it. Retirement options have to be considered."

Other respondents recommended that programs maintain good linkages with local elder services. Indeed, 74% of the programs had accessed generic senior services for some of their residents, the highest percentage for any community residential type. For example, one program was located in a public housing project for the elderly that was also mandated to serve handicapped persons. This program said that the arrangement has been "ideal for these clients."

Another common programmatic issue expressed by these programs was the lack of day program options. As one respondent put it, "I worry that there aren't enough options for people who might choose not to work. Some of our clients don't see seniors programs as desirable. Right now they are working, but if they stop, there really aren't other alternatives."

The average apartment program served 4.1 residents, of whom an average of 3.4 were age 55 or over. A little more than half (53%) served some residents who were under age 55. The average age of the residents was 61.1 years. Almost all of the elderly mentally retarded residents were either mildly retarded (48%) or moderately retarded (45%). The majority (59%) of these residents were male.

While only 5% of the elderly mentally retarded residents were described as being in excellent health given their age and disabilities, almost two-thirds (64%) were said to be in good health. About a quarter (23%) were in fair health, and the remainder (8%) were described as being in poor health.

The majority (59%) of the elderly mentally retarded residents attended sheltered workshops or vocational programs during the day. Nine percent attended day activity programs for mentally retarded persons of all ages, while another 9% attended generic senior citizen programs. A small percentage attended special day programs for older mentally retarded persons (6%), had no formal day program and remained at the residence during the day (7%), or attended other types of programs (10%).

In sum, apartment programs serving elderly mentally retarded persons were comparatively small programs that provided a modest number of services to the residents. They served the highest percentage of mildly retarded individuals of any residential type in the National Survey. Virtually all of the residents were still involved in formal day programs, although a frequent concern of programs was the lack of alternatives should the current day programs no longer be appropriate. Interestingly, these programs were the most likely of any residential type to have accessed generic senior citizen programs on behalf of their older residents.

Mixed Residential Programs

This category includes residential programs that serve multiple target populations. Mentally retarded persons constituted an average of only 46% of the total clients served. Other types of residents served included nonhandicapped older persons, persons with a history of mental illness or emotional problems, or persons with physical handicaps. Twenty such programs located in 8 states were included in the National Survey.

About one-third (30%) of these programs were individually operated proprietary programs, while one-fifth (20%) were sponsored by private nonprofit agencies. The majority described their location as rural (55%). Not surprisingly, less than half (40%) were originally started to serve older mentally retarded persons.

These were among the oldest programs in the National Survey, with the average year in which the first mentally retarded person over age 55 was served being 1977. They were also the least expensive program model, with an average per resident budget of $5,224 in 1984. There were an average of 4.9 residents for each staff person in these programs (comparable to the foster homes described earlier). Interestingly, over half of these programs reported employing a nurse. Less than a fifth had other types of professional staff employed. Just over half (55%) of the programs reported that staff had received special training in the care of older mentally retarded persons.

These programs were the least likely of any of the residential types to see elderly mentally retarded persons as having special needs (only 6% of the programs). As one respondent stated, "You need to treat the elderly mentally retarded persons as you would any elderly person. Both need love and attention."

The average number of services provided in these programs was 8.9, the third lowest among the types. These were not, in general, residences that provided training or therapeutic services to clients. Rather, these homes often described themselves as "retirement" homes and were more oriented towards social, recreational, and leisure activities than towards individualized goal planning. For example, one respondent noted that she was "starting a crafts program in the house and bringing in outside volunteers to help get it going. We also have lots of children come visit and bring their pets. They're really well received."

Mixed residential programs were the largest of the residential types, with an average size of 29.5 clients, 8.6 of whom were elderly mentally retarded residents. The average age of all residents was 63.7 years.

Most of the elderly mentally retarded clients served were mildly (40%) or moderately (51%) retarded. Nine percent were either severely or profoundly retarded. The majority (70%) were described as being in good health. One-fifth (20%) were described as being in fair health with the remaining described as being in either excellent (7%) or poor (3%) health.

Over half (55%) of the elderly mentally retarded persons living in these homes were not involved in formal day programs and spent their days at the residence; no other residential model had such a high percentage of its residents remaining at home during the day. While 2%

attended senior citizens programs, none went to special day programs for mentally retarded elders.

In sum, mixed residential programs were typically large programs that provided a moderate amount of personal and social services to their residents. These programs were among the oldest of the residential types and were often serving mentally retarded elders along with nonretarded elders. There was a lower percentage of respondents who saw their mentally retarded elders as having specialized needs. There was a marked informality about these residences—most of the residents spent their days at home engaged in a variety of leisure activities.

COMPARISONS ACROSS MODELS

Salient differences among the residential models were analyzed using one way analyses of variance. Our purpose was to expose both similarities and differences in program types serving elderly mentally retarded persons in order to highlight the major organizational, programmatic, and client characteristics that may guide future planning and development in the residential care system.

Organizational Context Variables

Table 5-3 presents the results of one-way analyses of variance where the residential typology is the independent variable and nine organizational variables are the dependent measures. Significant differences among the residential models were found with respect to each of the organizational characteristics analyzed. Apartment programs were the most likely to be sponsored by a private nonprofit agency, while foster homes were the least likely. Group homes with nurses were the most likely to be sponsored by multiprogram agencies, and mixed residential programs were the most likely to be the single program offered by the operator.

Differences were found regarding the ages of the programs (based on the average year that the program model first started serving elderly mentally retarded persons): mixed residential and foster home programs were the oldest, while apartment programs were the most recently started. ICFs/MR were the most likely and group homes the least likely to have been intentionally created to serve elderly mentally retarded persons.

There were significant differences in geographic location. While foster homes and group homes with nurses were rarely located in urban areas, at least a third of the programs in the other residential types were urban programs.

TABLE 5-3

Mean Values for Organizational Context Variables by Community Residential Program Typology (N = 186)

VARIABLE	FOSTER HOMES (n = 26)	GROUP HOMES (n = 50)	GROUP HOMES WITH NURSES (n = 27)	ICFS/ MR (n = 44)	APART- MENT PRO- GRAMS (n = 19)	MIXED RESI- DENTIAL (n = 20)	F
A. *Sponsoring program*							
1. Private nonprofit[a]	.12	.60	.52	.55	.90	.20	8.88***
2. Multiprogram agency[a]	.44	.92	.96	.89	.95	.25	20.51***
3. Agency sponsors other MR programs[a]	.58	.89	.81	.87	.89	.05	1.57
4. Agency sponsors aging (non-MR) programs[a]	.42	.20	.27	.21	.33	.60	1.34
B. *Program history and location*							
1. Year first served elderly mentally retarded persons (EMR)	1977	1981	1980	1981	1982	1977	5.53***
2. Created to serve EMR	.46	.34	.41	.71	.37	.40	3.09***
3. In urban location[a]	.15	.43	.11	.42	.37	.35	2.76*
C. *Program resources*							
1. 1984 per client budget	$5,474	$15,240	$22,089	$30,773	$15,619	$5,224	2.85**
2. Number of different sources	2.35	3.00	3.41	3.09	2.00	2.95	3.88**
3. Received special grants — first year[a]	.00	.28	.30	.23	.42	.05	3.58**
4. Received special grants — ever[a]	.00	.36	.30	.23	.47	.11	4.17**

[a] Coded as 0 = no   1 = yes
* = p<.05.   ** = p<.01.   *** = p<.001

The 1984 per client budgets ranged from a low of $5,224 for mixed residential programs to a high of $30,773 for ICF/MR programs. Interestingly, there was on average nearly a $7,000 difference in the per client budgets of group homes as compared with budgets of group homes with nurses. Programs averaged between two and three different sources of funds to support their programs. Special grants were more likely to have been received by apartment programs and group homes than the other residential categories.

Program Characteristic Variables

Table 5-4 presents the results of analyses of variance in which the residential typology was the independent variable and program characteristics were the dependent measures. As shown in this table, there were

TABLE 5-4

Program Characteristic Variables by Community Residential
Program Typology ($N = 186$)

VARIABLE	FOSTER HOMES ($n = 26$)	GROUP HOMES ($n = 50$)	GROUP HOMES WITH NURSES ($n = 27$)	ICFS/ MR ($n = 44$)	APART- MENT PRO- GRAMS ($n = 19$)	MIXED RESI- DENTIAL ($n = 20$)	F
A. *Size*							
1. Mean number of total residents	3.65	6.88	8.85	17.02	4.05	29.50	20.47***
2. Mean number of EMR residents	3.19	5.37	6.31	13.43	3.37	8.60	10.62***
3. Percent EMR residents	90	80	74	80	82	32	23.30**
B. *Staffing*							
1. Mean number of total staff	1.65	4.20	6.75	15.28	4.23	7.20	18.86***
2. Mean number of residents per one staff person	5.50	1.81	1.34	1.32	1.64	4.86	7.59***
3. Percent of programs with:							
a. Administrators	69	98	96	100	79	100	7.81***
b. Direct care staff	65	98	96	100	84	90	7.32***
c. Nurses	8	0	100	100	5	55	166.78***
d. Physicians	0	0	4	25	0	10	6.32***
e. Therapists (PT, OT)	0	2	0	43	0	15	14.65***
f. Psychologists	0	2	33	48	0	0	15.79***
g. Social workers	15	26	48	66	16	5	9.30***
h. Homemakers	4	2	4	25	5	35	5.94***
i. Teachers	0	16	4	11	21	0	2.32*
4. Percent programs providing staff training on aging	62	58	59	88	47	55	3.09*
5. Percent programs recommending staff training on:							
a. Generic seniors programs	10	38	27	14	20	22	.72
b. Biological aspects of aging	30	76	91	57	30	56	3.30**
c. Psychological aspects of aging	20	48	46	29	20	44	.83
C. *Services*							
1. Number of services to EMR residents	4.9	9.7	12.4	15.8	8.3	8.9	31.87***
2. Number of services to nonelderly MR	5.0	9.2	11.8	15.3	7.9	8.7	25.08***
3. Number of health services	.4	.8	2.2	2.6	.6	1.6	42.61***
a. Percent providing medical	8	0	26	41	0	20	8.57***
b. Percent providing dental	0	2	19	21	0	5	3.99**
c. Percent providing nursing	15	36	100	100	11	65	11.21***
d. Percent providing nutrition	19	57	85	98	53	65	14.26***

TABLE 5-4

Program Characteristic Variables by Community Residential Program Typology ($N = 186$) (Continued)

VARIABLE	FOSTER HOMES ($n = 26$)	GROUP HOMES ($n = 50$)	GROUP HOMES WITH NURSES ($n = 27$)	ICFS/ MR ($n = 44$)	APART- MENT PRO- GRAMS ($n = 19$)	MIXED RESI- DENTIAL ($n = 20$)	F
C. *Services* (Continued)							
4. Number of therapeutic services	.4	.9	1.6	2.8	.5	.8	27.91***
a. Percent providing PT or OT	4	8	22	66	5	10	18.24***
b. Percent providing speech	0	8	19	57	0	10	15.36***
c. Percent providing psychological	8	12	41	68	0	20	15.70***
d. Percent providing social work	27	66	82	84	42	35	8.78***
5. Number of support services	1.5	2.8	3.0	3.1	2.5	2.2	14.14***
a. Percent providing transportation	58	92	100	100	74	80	8.50***
b. Percent providing financial assistance	23	72	70	86	63	30	9.78***
c. Percent providing legal assistance	4	26	26	23	16	5	1.93
d. Percent providing recreational	69	92	100	100	95	100	6.82***
6. Number of social services	.7	1.4	1.2	1.4	1.3	.9	8.88***
a. Percent providing adult education	0	38	22	41	47	15	4.57***
b. Percent providing self care	65	98	96	96	84	75	5.88***
7. Percent utilizing generic seniors programs	39	64	56	57	74	50	1.46
8. Seniors centers staff receptivity rating[a]	2.80	2.58	2.53	2.40	2.29	2.80	1.48
9. Seniors centers client receptivity rating[a]	2.40	2.42	2.40	2.36	2.25	2.60	.35

[a] Rating scale: $1 =$ not at all receptive $2 =$ somewhat receptive $3 =$ very receptive
* $= p<.05$.   ** $= p<.01$.   *** $= p<.001$.

significant differences in the size of the programs, with mixed residential programs averaging almost 30 residents per program as compared with not quite 4 residents each for foster homes. Further, the program types differed in the percentage of residents who were elderly mentally retarded persons. Less than a third of the mixed residential programs' residents were elderly mentally retarded persons, compared with over 80% for foster homes, group homes, apartment programs, and ICFs/MR.

There were significant differences in the resident-to-staff ratios among the programs. Foster homes and mixed residential programs had the most residents per staff, while each of the other models approached a 1:1 ratio. There were also significant differences with respect to the percentage of programs that employed both direct care staff and various types of professional staff. In general, ICFs/MR and group homes with nurses were the most frequent employers of nurses, psychologists, and social workers. Foster homes were the least professionalized of the residential models.

Except for apartment programs, at least half of the programs within each type provided some staff training on aging and mental retardation. Respondents from group homes and group homes with nurses were the most likely to recommend that staff receive training in the biological aspects of aging.

There were significant differences in the average number of services provided among the residential types. The ICFs/MR and group homes with nurses program types were the most service-intensive models, while foster homes were the least service oriented. The differences in amount and type of service provision were primarily attributable to the extent to which nursing and therapeutic services were provided.

There were no significant differences among the various types in the percentage of programs that had accessed senior citizens services for their residents. Further, in all program models, respondents rated the staff in the senior citizen programs as slightly more receptive to participation of elderly mentally retarded persons than the nonretarded clients served.

Resident Characteristic Variables

Table 5-5 presents the results of the analyses of variance in which the resident characteristics served as the dependent measures and the residential typology as the independent variable. Significant differences among program models were found with respect to the average age of the residents, which ranged from 58.7 (for group homes with nurses) to 65.9 years (for foster homes). Significant differences were also found for the percentage of residents in the 70 and over age category. Mixed residential homes had the highest percentage of such residents (37%), while apartment programs had the lowest (12%). Interestingly, mixed residential programs (which had the highest average age for the program's oldest resident) also had the lowest average age for the program's youngest resident (34.35 years). The spread in average ages for the youngest and oldest residents in the program was also the most dramatic in this residential type.

While the differences were not significant, a higher percentage of

TABLE 5-5

Resident Characteristic Variables by Community
Residential Typology (*N* = 186)

VARIABLE[a]	FOSTER HOMES (*n* = 26)	GROUP HOMES (*n* = 50)	GROUP HOMES WITH NURSES (*n* = 27)	ICFS/ MR (*n* = 44)	APART-MENT PRO-GRAMS (*n* = 19)	MIXED RESI-DENTIAL (*n* = 20)	F
A. *Age*							
1. Average age (in years)	65.91	61.85	58.68	62.56	61.05	63.69	3.16**
2. Percent below 22	0	0	0	0	0	1	3.12**
3. Percent aged 22–50	5	15	17	14	7	14	2.54*
4. Percent aged 51–54	5	5	9	6	12	8	1.07
5. Percent aged 55–60	21	23	30	22	31	13	2.05
6. Percent aged 61–69	39	33	30	31	38	27	.93
7. Percent aged 70 +	30	24	14	27	12	37	3.86**
8. Average age of youngest resident	56.65	47.74	42.74	45.52	53.26	34.35	11.10***
9. Average age of oldest resident	71.65	72.84	70.70	77.16	66.95	85.45	16.66***
B. *Gender*							
1. Percent female	64	53	45	52	41	43	1.29
C. *Level of retardation*							
1. Average level of MR[b]	1.12	1.16	1.06	.86	1.41	1.30	3.95**
2. Percentage mild	33	40	32	28	48	40	1.34
3. Percentage moderate	47	37	43	30	45	51	1.64
4. Percentage severe/ profound	20	23	25	42	7	9	6.12***
D. *Health*							
1. Average health status[c]	1.91	1.91	1.94	1.92	1.66	1.81	.77
2. Percent excellent health	26	24	26	20	5	7	2.11
3. Percent good health	44	51	45	55	64	70	1.99
4. Percent fair health	25	18	23	21	23	20	.28
5. Percent poor health	5	7	6	4	8	3	.44
E. *Day placements*							
1. Percent in special programs for EMR residents	4	18	14	15	6	0	1.70
2. Percent in senior citizen programs	14	10	1	5	9	2	1.62
3. Percent in vocational program	7	28	33	24	59	9	6.76***
4. Percent day activity program	17	21	19	8	9	22	.36
5. Percent in residence— formal program	4	8	14	30	0	10	4.31**
6. Percent in residence— no formal program	48	5	12	7	7	55	14.59***
7. Percent in other programs	6	10	7	11	10	2	.66

[a] The unit of analysis for variables in Section A is the total resident group in each setting. The unit of analysis in Sections B through E is the elderly mentally retarded group in each setting. [b] Coded as 2 = mild 1 = moderate 0 = severe or profound [c] Coded as: 3 = excellent 2 = good 1 = fair 0 = poor, per judgments of the respondents
* $p < .05$. ** $p < .01$. *** $p < .001$.

foster home residents were women than in any other residential category. Apartment program residents were the most likely to be male.

Significant differences among types were found with respect to the average level of retardation of residents, with ICFs/MR having the most cognitively impaired residents and apartment programs having the least cognitively impaired residents. There were no significant differences regarding the health status of elderly mentally retarded persons in various residential programs, and in no type of program were more than half the residents rated in either fair or poor health.

With respect to day placements, there were significant differences for the percentage of residents who attended vocational programs (apartment programs having the highest and foster homes having the lowest), who stayed at home but engaged in formal day programs (with ICFs/MR having the highest and apartment programs having none), and who stayed at home with no formal programs (with mixed residential and foster homes both having at least half their residents at home and group homes having the lowest percentage of residents so occupied).

CONCLUSIONS

This chapter has described 186 community-based programs in which approximately 1,350 elderly mentally retarded persons lived. From these programs, six distinct types were identified. While the initial typology was developed on the basis of a qualitative content analysis of each residential program, the utility of the typology was subsequently confirmed through quantitative analyses that found significant differences among the models on a host of organizational, programmatic, and client characteristic variables. The identified types paralleled existing residential typologies with one exception: group homes with nurses were distinguished as a separate model because they represent an important modification of traditional staffing patterns of group homes.

Mixed residential programs had the greatest number of distinctive features among the residential typology. These programs were among the oldest, served the largest number of clients, had the lowest percentage of elderly mentally retarded persons compared with the total client group, provided among the lowest average number of services, had the highest percentage of residents at home during the day with no formal programs, and consequently were the least expensive of the models. These programs were the least likely to see elderly mentally retarded persons as having special needs. Rather the programs tended to be very informal both structurally and programmatically.

At the other extreme, ICFs/MR had both the structural and programmatic capacity to meet the needs of very challenging residents.

More residences in this model were specifically designed to meet the needs of elderly mentally retarded persons than in any other category. They served the highest percentage of severely and profoundly retarded residents, had the lowest resident-to-staff ratio, provided the largest number of services, were the most likely to have a high percentage of their residents in some type of formal day program, and were consequently the most costly of the residential models.

Group homes with nurses stood between the highly professionalized and service oriented ICF/MR programs and the traditionally staffed group homes. A higher percentage of group homes with nurses were specifically designed to serve elderly mentally retarded persons than was true for group homes without nurses. Further, group homes with nurses had a higher per client budget, lower resident-to-staff ratios, higher average number of services, larger program size, slightly higher percentage of severely and profoundly retarded elderly residents, and yet lower average age than was true for traditional group homes.

The apartment programs had several key features: they were more likely to access generic senior services, provided more protective oversight than formal services to the residents, were very unlikely to have residents stay home during the day, and served more mildly retarded residents than did the other program model. They were, therefore, structurally and programmatically less likely to be as adaptable to the changing (and intensifying) health, emotional, and social needs of mentally retarded persons as they aged. Indeed, the very nature of apartment programs—with their more varied and less intensive staffing patterns—suggests that these programs may well be suitable for older mentally retarded persons who are still capable of a high level of independent functioning. Their capacity to serve elders who are declining in emotional and physical stamina remains unknown.

This discussion suggests that existing community-based residential models have demonstrated a capacity to adapt their structures and programs to serve elderly mentally retarded persons. Group homes, perhaps the most deeply rooted of the community-based residential models in the field of mental retardation, have further shown an ability to modify their staffing structure (by the inclusion of a program nurse) as one mechanism for meeting the needs of a specific target group. As discussed in Chapter 4 and earlier in this chapter, almost half of the community residential programs described themselves as having evolved into the care of elderly mentally retarded persons. The elasticity of the community residential care system for mentally retarded persons, as illustrated by the ways in which service delivery and staffing patterns have been modified, is quite remarkable.

The enthusiasm and dedication of the staff in these programs deserves special mention. While not a quantifiable characteristic (at least in the present study), the depth of concern, commitment, and attachment of staff to their residents was a thread woven throughout the informal remarks offered during scores of interviews conducted across the country. It expressed itself in the common refrain from respondents that adequate retirement programs were lacking, that too often residents' medical needs were not well met, that staff needed a better understanding of the gradual changes seen in residents, and that more resources are needed to enrich the lives of the residents.

Many of the problems articulated by staff are not unique to programs for elderly mentally retarded persons. What was impressive, however, was the pioneering spirit of the staff charged with their care. The curiosity of the respondents regarding this study and its potential impact on the programs they offer attested to their need for both sharing with and learning from other programs. The vast majority of the programs participating in the National Survey conveyed an enthusiasm and energy for their work with elderly mentally retarded persons that warrants particular notice.

Chapter 6

Community-Based
Day Programs

The purpose of this chapter is to present descriptive information about the 135 community-based day programs that participated in the National Survey. A typology was developed consisting of five distinct models of day program service delivery. Each of these models will be described by means of quantitative and qualitative data.

BACKGROUND

Janicki, Otis, Puccio, Rettig, and Jacobson (1985) noted that "in the broadest sense, the service needs of older developmentally disabled persons are similar to those of younger developmentally disabled persons and other older, but non-disabled persons" (p. 292). As we discussed in Chapter 2, past research has indicated both similarities and differences in the characteristics and service needs of elderly mentally retarded persons and each of their two reference groups (i.e., younger mentally retarded adults and elderly nondisabled persons). It is not clear from the available research whether elderly mentally retarded persons would benefit most from day programs designed for younger mentally retarded adults, from day programs for nonretarded senior citizens, or from a combination of the two.

A variety of types of day programs exist for mentally retarded persons, while different types of day programs have been developed for nonretarded elderly persons. White, Hill, Lakin, and Bruininks (1984) described four types of day placements for mentally retarded persons: public and private school; vocational, work, or training programs; day activity centers; and home-based training by outside staff. In their 1982 national probability sample of mentally retarded persons who lived in residential facilities, the day placements of those aged 65 and older were reported. The majority of the elderly residents of community residential facilities (76%) and of those who lived in public residential facilities (61%) had no day placement. In both of these samples, the most common day placement of those elders who left the residential unit during the day was the day activity center. No descriptive data were available about the characteristics of day activity centers that served elderly mentally retarded persons.

Janicki and MacEachron (1984) reported the results of a statewide needs assessment of older developmentally disabled adults in New York state conducted between 1978 and 1982. They divided the sample into three groups: late middle aged (53–62), aging (63–72), and aged (73–99). The proportion of sample members who had no day activity increased with advancing age (12%, 14%, and 20%, respectively), as did the proportion who received therapeutic activities in their places of residence (32%, 34%, and 46%, respectively). Conversely, the proportion who participated in sheltered workshops or day habilitation training decreased with advancing age (32%, 27%, and 12% and 12%, 12%, and 10%, respectively). Fewer than 5% in any age group attended senior citizens programs.

Senior citizens day programs can be categorized as either multipurpose senior centers or adult day care centers. Multipurpose senior centers have been defined as "a single setting in which older people can take part in social activities as well as have access to essential services (including) nutrition, health, employment, transportation, social work and other supportive services, education, creative arts, recreation and leadership, and volunteer opportunities" (Lowy, 1985b, p. 274). Also according to Lowy (1985b), there are currently over 8,000 centers in the United States serving approximately 8 million elders. Of particular relevance in this context, fully 84% of the centers serve some chronically ill, frail, or physically or mentally impaired elders. Lowy (1985b) identified the following two issues currently facing senior centers: the extent to which the dominant program emphasis should shift from education/recreation to treatment; and the extent to which impaired elders should be included with nonimpaired elders. The receptivity of multipurpose seniors centers to elderly mentally retarded persons will depend in large part on how these two issues are resolved.

An adult day care center has been defined as a "program that provides a gamut of services in a congregate setting, enhancing the daily lives of its participants and supporting their continued involvement in the community. Adult day care is a generic term that applies to a variety of programs offering services that range from active rehabilitation to social and health related care . . ." (National Institute of Adult Day Care, 1982). In 1982, there were an estimated 800 adult day care centers in the United States serving approximately 20,000 elders (National Institute of Adult Day Care, 1982).

Robins (1981) classified adult day care centers into three types: restoration programs, offering intensive one-on-one health supportive services by certified therapeutic specialists; maintenance programs, offering health monitoring, supervised therapeutic individual and group activities, and psychosocial services; and social programs, offering socialization, hot lunches, transportation, and health maintenance. Huttman (1985) offered a somewhat different typology: medical day care centers, which provide medical and rehabilitative services to persons recovering from acute illnesses and who need intensive rehabilitation or to chronically ill persons needing continued health supports; general social day care centers, which provide functionally impaired but cognitively intact elders with a social experience; and social day care for cognitively impaired elders, which provide social experiences to elders with psychiatric problems or dementia (including Alzheimer's disease). The first of these three types can be certified by Medicaid as an adult day health care center if federal regulations are met, while the latter two types are generally not Medicaid certified. According to Huttman (1985), more than 50% of existing adult day care centers are general social day care centers, while there are very few social day care centers for cognitively impaired elders. The extent to which mentally retarded elders participate in the various types of adult day care centers has not yet been reported in the literature.

THE DAY PROGRAM TYPOLOGY

In the context of the limited available research on day programs for elderly mentally retarded persons, the National Survey included questions specifically about day programs. On the basis of a qualitative analysis of the responses to these questions, a typology of community-based day programs was developed. Table 6-1 presents the distribution of the 135 community-based day programs across the five types of programs and a list of defining characteristics of each type.

The remainder of this chapter includes two sections. The first presents an overview of each of the five types of community-based day programs, including descriptive data and case examples. The second presents a statistical comparison of these types with the objective of identifying specific characteristics and dimensions that differentiate each from the others.

Vocational Day Activity Programs

A vocational day activity program is a full-time program for elderly mentally retarded adults in which vocational activities are included in the program of services. The 35 vocational day activity programs in the National Survey were located in 18 states.

TABLE 6-1

Typology of Community-Based Day Programs (*N* = 135)

TYPE	*n*	PERCENT	CHARACTERISTICS
Vocational day activity program	35	25.9	—MR program —Full time (21 hours/wk or more) —Some vocational component
Day activity program	37	27.4	—MR program —Full time (21 hours/wk or more) —No vocational component
Supplemental retirement program	30	22.2	—MR program —Not full time (less than 21 hours/wk) —No vocational services —Center based
Leisure and outreach services	17	12.6	—MR program —Not full time and atypical scheduling —Not a regular day program (e.g., summer camps, courses, community outreach —May not be center based
Senior citizens program	16	11.9	—Not a MR program —Primarily serves elderly nondisabled or disabled nonretarded elders —Center based
TOTAL	135	100.0	

Vocational day activity programs are the most similar of the five models in the day program typology to traditional day programs for mentally retarded adults. These programs are often operated by agencies that also sponsor sheltered workshops and day activity centers. Such agencies have recognized the special needs that emerge when mentally retarded persons age and have designed vocational day activity programs in response to these perceived needs. For example, one program director explained that "clients are transferred from the sheltered workshop to the Older Adult program when they fall behind in vocational production. The Older Adult Program is an *alternative* to retirement, not a retirement option." It was common for respondents to note that they decided to continue to provide active treatment to elders who participated in vocational day activity programs because of funding requirements from clients' residential settings.

On the average, vocational day activity programs began serving elderly mentally retarded persons in 1981. Fewer than half (43%) of these programs were created specifically for the purpose of serving elderly mentally retarded persons. Instead, in the majority of programs the decision was made to modify existing services because a critical mass of their clients had reached old age. Vocational day activity programs served an average of 20.12 clients of whom 13.64 were over the age of 55. The average per client budget in 1984 was $6,558.19, the second highest in the typology.

There was one full-time staff member (FTE) for every 5.49 clients in vocational day activity programs. Half of these programs had therapists (occupational and/or physical therapists) on staff, a higher percentage than in the other four models. The percentage of programs with teachers (35%) was also higher than in the other models, reflecting the goals and structure of the services in such programs. Fully 83% of the vocational day activity programs provided special training to staff on aging, again a higher percentage than in any other model in the typology.

Vocational day activity programs tended to offer highly structured services. One staff member wrote: "Daily work assignments consist of food preparation and serving, dishwashing, bussing tables, general housekeeping and child care services offered to the preschool program . . . These work opportunities provide a means whereby each individual can earn a wage, thus providing funds for personal needs and community activities." Several programs noted that the pacing of activities had to be slower for the elderly clients than for the younger adult clients served by the sponsoring agency. For example, the director of one program noted that: "These clients need much more time to do each thing. They need 15 minutes to put on their coats and get out to the vans. Also, relaxation time needs to be built in."

The clients in vocational day activity programs averaged 60.14 years of age, the youngest average age among the models in the typology. Only 47% of these clients were female, a smaller percentage than in any other model. Further, these clients were judged to be the most intellectually impaired; fully 42% of the clients served in these programs were severely or profoundly retarded. Staff perceived large differences between the elderly mentally retarded clients and the younger retarded clients they served in terms of their energy levels and memory and reported that these perceived differences had an impact on the kinds of activities provided to the elderly clients. Clients in vocational day activity programs tended to live in group homes (40%), foster homes (13%), ICFs/MR (12%), and nursing homes (11%) in addition to other residential settings.

In sum, vocational day activity programs were modifications of traditional day programs that aimed to forestall retirement for elderly mentally retarded persons. As the clients in this type of program tended to be the youngest among the models in the day program typology, this service type may be the first option used when an older mentally retarded person's functional abilities begin to decline.

Day Activity Programs

A day activity program is a full-time program for mentally retarded adults in which no vocational services are provided. While the 37 day activity programs in the National Survey were located in 13 states, nearly half ($n = 18$, 48.6%) were in New York state alone.

These programs were among the most recently developed of the models in the typology. Half (51%) were created specifically for the purpose of serving elderly mentally retarded persons, while the other half evolved into this type of program as clients aged. The agencies that operated day activity programs were largely private nonprofit corporations (73%). Very few also sponsored generic senior citizens programs (only 14%, the second lowest percentage among the models in the typology). The day activity programs in the National Survey served an average of 19.57 clients, of whom 16.00 were elderly mentally retarded persons. The 1984 annual per client budget of $7,433.43 was highest among the models. Over a third (36%) received special grant funds to serve elderly mentally retarded clients.

Philosophically, these programs aimed to provide a normalized retirement option for mentally retarded elders. One program director noted that "this program has been organized to replicate senior citizens group activities normally found in the community." Another explained that the goal of the program was to offer the possibility of retirement, which was operationalized to mean more choice, less structure, and less intense programming. These tended to be self-contained programs with a relatively low level of physical and social integration with younger retarded or nonretarded elderly persons than in the other models. Interestingly, staff from day activity programs were more likely than staff from other models to know of other programs that served elderly mentally retarded persons (51%).

The clients in day activity programs averaged 63.64 years of age. Almost two-thirds were female, the second highest percentage in the day program typology. Overall, their average level of functioning was second lowest, with only 28% mildly retarded, 35% moderately retarded, and fully 37% severely or profoundly retarded. In contrast with vocational day activity programs, a higher percentage of day activity program clients lived in foster homes (19%) and in ICFs/MR (23%, the highest frequency in the sample) and a smaller percentage lived in group homes (30%).

One program described its admission policy as seeking "multiply handicapped retarded persons aged 60 or older who need retirement in place of a vocational placement." In order for an applicant to be accepted into this program, regression in skills had to be demonstrated and evidence that the client could benefit from a lower stress, slower paced recreational activity had to be presented. This profile typified the goals, content, and structure of day activity programs for elderly mentally retarded adults.

Supplemental Retirement Programs

A supplemental retirement program is a part-time day program for mentally retarded elders. The focus was on recreational rather than vocational activities, and most programs clearly articulated that a major objective was to provide a retirement option. The reduction in hours from full time to part time was seen as a response to the reduced capacity of clients to participate in a full-day program. The 30 supplemental retirement programs in the National Survey were located in 15 states.

On the average, supplemental retirement programs began operation in 1980. The programs in this model can be characterized as intentionally planned and innovative. Fully 77% were developed specifically for the purpose of providing day services to elderly mentally retarded adults, the highest percentage in the typology. These programs also were more likely than other models to have received special grants for providing services to elderly mentally retarded persons during their first year of operation (37%). The annual per client budget in 1984 was $4,483.13.

The average program served 19.47 clients, most of whom (88%) were over the age of 55. The staff to client ratio was lower than in the two full-time program models, with one staff member for every 8.89 clients. In addition to direct care staff, 33% of the programs had therapists (occupational and/or physical therapists) on staff and 37% had social workers. Only 10% of the supplemental retirement programs employed nurses.

Consistent with the name of this model, retirement was a major theme expressed by staff. One program director noted, "Age has given our clients a right to make choices." The range of activities provided in these retirement programs was noteworthy. For example, one program listed the following:

— Volunteer work	— Rug hooking
— Gardening	— Woodworking
— Bowling	— Ceramics
— Arts and crafts	— Assertiveness training
— Cooking	— Participating in the local
— Sewing	senior center
— Music	

A staff member from another program, which met for 10 hours each week, explained: "Our program provides these older adults with an opportunity to engage in a wide variety of community activities, such as swimming, bowling, movies, restaurants, library, parks, trips to the city, classes in ceramics, yoga, chorus . . ."

While community participation was a widely articulated theme, these programs were center based, with space set aside for staff and clients; the center served as a home base for community participation. These programs had a higher rate of physical and social integration with younger mentally retarded adults and with elderly nonretarded persons than three of the other models in the typology (the exception was senior citizens programs), and they were the most likely of the four programs designed for mentally retarded persons in the typology to use generic services for senior citizens for their own clients (77%).

Staff from supplemental retirement programs were the most likely to view elderly mentally retarded persons as having special needs (97% of the programs in this model). They were also more likely than staff from the other types of day programs to report differences between elderly mentally retarded clients and their younger retarded adults in the following specific areas: service needs (72% reported this difference), skill level (55%), motivational level (52%), and emotional needs (48%). Similarly, staff from supplemental retirement programs were more likely than staff from the other types of programs to be concerned about clients' medical problems (90% reported this concern), providing a quality retirement option for the (80%), dealing with the death of clients or their relatives (70%), and the need for guardianship (37%). Somewhat paradoxically in light of the intensity of their concern and commitment, staff from these programs gave their programs the lowest ratings of any model as to how well their services were meeting clients' needs.

The clients in supplemental retirement programs averaged 62.99 years of age. More than half (57%) were female. They were about average for the sample of day programs in level of retardation (33% mild, 43% moderate, 24% severe or profound), but had a higher percentage of clients reportedly in poor health (12%) of all the day program models. A large proportion of the clients lived in group homes (45%), with foster homes and ICF/MR programs also frequently represented (13% and 15%, respectively).

The noteworthy aspect of supplemental retirement programs is that staff were less satisfied with the services they were providing and felt the clients had more special needs while in fact, with the exception of poorer health status, the clients did not seem to possess unusual characteristics. This seeming contradiction may be explained by the possibility that these staff had higher expectations and a higher level of investment in providing special services to elderly mentally retarded persons and that their standards were therefore more stringent.

Leisure and Outreach Services

This category includes a heterogeneous group of programs, all of which are part time, primarily serving mentally retarded elders, atypical in scheduling, and focused on leisure activities and/or community participation. Programs included in this model ranged from summer camps to in-home services to adult education classes to community outings. Clients spent an average of 10.48 hours per week at the program, less time than in any other model.

All 17 of the leisure and outreach programs, which were located in nine states, had served elderly mentally retarded persons since their inception. Nearly all (93%) of these programs were operated by agencies that sponsored other programs for mentally retarded persons. Very few agencies (13%) sponsored programs for nonretarded elders. Leisure and outreach programs were the least likely to use generic senior citizens services for their clients (only 50% did) and to integrate elderly nonretarded clients into their programs. Thus, this model was the least integrated with the aging services network.

The 1984 annual per client budget of $1,479.53 was by far the lowest in the day program sample. The number of budget sources was also smallest in this model. The staff to resident ratio was the poorest in the day program sample, with one staff member for every 9.84 clients. Staff in leisure and outreach programs were less likely than staff in any other day program model to have received special training on aging and mental retardation. Only about 30% of these programs had social workers on staff and fewer than 20% had therapists or teachers. Only one program had a psychologist and one a nurse.

Few generalizations can be applied to leisure and outreach programs. One program consisted exclusively of field trips in the community, as its primary goal was increasing community participation and awareness for elderly mentally retarded persons. Each client in this program was accompanied by a nonretarded elder who volunteered for this program. Another program had three units of service: small group activities conducted by day program staff in the residential setting, one-on-one community outings, and group outings. Yet another program offered the following courses:

- Hobby shop
- Leisure counseling
- Tai Chi
- World Watch
- Bingo

- Yoga
- Bridge
- Nutrition
- Exercise
- Cooking

As noted above, this day program model also included camps in which mentally retarded elders were provided with "a normalized vacation experience where they can go to a resort, like anyone else." Finally, day and overnight respite care were included in some programs in this category.

The clients who participated in leisure and outreach services tended to be the highest functioning of any model in the day program typology, with fully 49% mildly retarded. These clients were also judged to be healthy, with 80% reportedly in good or excellent health. They averaged 63.79 years of age and more than half were female (55%). A higher proportion of clients in this type of program lived in group homes (51%) than in any of the other four types of day programs.

Leisure and outreach programs offered a wide variety of creative services to elderly mentally retarded persons at a comparatively low cost. These programs also provided a particularly important service to families through respite and in-home support. Further, given the variety of activities and services offered, the potential for leisure and outreach programs to provide individualized services tailored to clients' own needs seemed high. It was surprising that so few of these programs used generic senior citizens services in light of the high functional level of the clients and the emphasis placed by many respondents on community participation.

Senior Citizens Programs

The senior citizens programs included in the National Survey met three inclusion criteria: at least 10% of the clients served in the program were mentally retarded; at least 50% of the mentally retarded clients were age 55 or older; and two or more elderly mentally retarded persons were served by the program. Thus, senior citizens programs that served one or only a few mentally retarded elders were not included in the National Survey. It was our intention to include programs in which mentally retarded elders would constitute a visible minority. In fact, the 16 senior citizens programs in the National Survey served an average of 34.56 clients per program, of whom 8.63 were elderly mentally retarded persons. These programs were located in nine states.

The 16 senior citizens programs in the National Survey can be further divided into two subtypes: those for disabled seniors ($n = 8$) and those for the general elderly population ($n = 8$). This distinction is consistent with the work of Huttman (1985), which was summarized at the beginning of this chapter. She distinguished between general social day care centers and social day care for impaired elders. While the client groups of these two types differ, we found them to be very similar programmatically and therefore included them in a single model.

On average, the senior citizens programs in the National Survey began operation in 1979, making them the oldest of the models in the day program typology. Fully 73% of the agencies that operated these programs also sponsored programs that primarily served mentally retarded persons. Thus, there was a high level of structural integration of the mental retardation and aging services networks in senior citizens programs that served elderly mentally retarded clients. Paralleling this structural integration was programmatic integration: these programs were the highest among the models in the day program typology in physical and social integration of their elderly mentally retarded clients with both nonretarded elders and younger retarded adults.

The majority (75%) of the sponsoring agencies were private nonprofit corporations. The 1984 per client annual budget was $3,765.54, lower than those for three of the other four day program models, yet these programs received their funding from an average of 2.94 different sources, the largest number of funding sources per program among the day program models. Senior citizens programs were the most likely of all day program models to have received private fees from clients, and while they were unlikely to have received special grants for serving elderly retarded persons during their first year of operation (19%), this type of program was the most likely to have received such a special grant at some point during their years of operation (44%). A higher proportion of senior citizens programs had nurses (73%) and social workers (47%) on staff than in any other model in the day program typology.

Senior citizens programs were generally not established for the purpose of serving elderly mentally retarded persons. However, respondents frequently emphasized the importance of providing services to this group. One explained that "elderly mentally retarded persons seem to get lost in the shuffle. Once they are out of the workshop, they need to be able to participate in programs in order to feel worthwhile." Another emphasized that "we are an alternative to sitting home." Somewhat surprisingly, senior citizens programs were least likely among the programs in the typology to report that elderly mentally retarded persons had special needs (21%). Rather, respondents commented on the similarity between the needs of the elderly mentally retarded clients and their elderly nonretarded clients. One program director noted that "the differences between elderly and younger mentally retarded persons parallel differences between the general population of elders and younger persons. They are both due to the issues of aging." Some programs reported that the two client groups had to get used to each other at first. "Acceptance of the developmentally disabled by the normal clients was an issue." Conversely, another program staffer noted that "we have to help our mentally retarded clients understand the erratic behavior and mood swings of our nonretarded clients with Alzheimer's disease."

The mentally retarded clients served in senior citizens programs averaged 66.38 years of age, the oldest group among the day program models. Almost two-thirds were female, the highest percentage in any day program model. Their functional level was second highest among day program models, with 44% mildly retarded, 38% moderately retarded, and only 18% severely or profoundly retarded. Their health was reportedly the most impaired, with fully 38% of the mentally retarded clients in senior citizens programs described as being in fair or poor health. Senior citizens programs were more likely than the other day program models to serve mentally retarded persons who lived with their families (14%) and in semi-independent apartments (7%).

The potential of senior citizens programs to serve elderly mentally retarded persons has only begun to be explored. One program director offered the following advice to other generic aging programs that might be interested in including mentally retarded elders: "It is important to have friends of one's own age, but don't assume a single solution because of age."

COMPARISONS ACROSS
MODELS

Organizational Context Variables

Table 6-2 presents the results of a series of one-way analyses of variance in which the day program typology was the independent variable and organizational context variables were the dependent variables.

As shown in Table 6-2 the majority of day programs were operated by private nonprofit agencies that also sponsored other programs. There were significant differences among the day program models with respect to the percentage of agencies that sponsored other programs for mentally retarded persons (vocational day activity programs being the highest and senior citizens programs the lowest) and with respect to the percentage of agencies that sponsored programs for nonretarded elders (senior citizens programs being the highest and leisure and outreach services the lowest).

While there were no significant differences among the day program models in the year that programs first served elderly mentally retarded clients (models varied between 1979 and 1981), the models did differ in the percentage of programs that were created specifically for the purpose of providing services for elderly mentally retarded persons. Supplemental

TABLE 6-2

Mean Values for Organizational Context Variables by Community Day
Program Typology (N = 135)

VARIABLE	VOCA-TIONAL DAY ACTIVITY (n = 35)	DAY ACTIVITY (n = 37)	SUPPLE-MENTAL RETIRE-MENT (n = 30)	LEISURE AND OUTREACH (n = 17)	SENIOR CITIZENS CENTERS (n = 16)	F
A. *Sponsoring Program*						
1. Private nonprofit[a]	0.77	0.73	0.57	0.47	0.75	1.84
2. Multiprogram agency[a]	1.00	0.97	1.00	0.88	0.94	1.82
3. Agency sponsors other MR programs[a]	1.00	0.86	0.97	0.93	0.73	3.23**
4. Agency sponsors aging (non-MR) programs[a]	0.23	0.14	0.30	0.13	0.60	3.67**
B. *Program History and Location*						
1. Year first served elderly mentally retarded	1981	1981	1980	1981	1979	0.79
2. Created to serve EMR[a]	0.43	0.51	0.77	0.65	0.25	3.82**
3. In urban location[a]	0.41	0.41	0.45	0.56	0.63	0.79
C. *Program Resources*						
1. 1984 per client budget	6558.19	7433.43	4483.13	1479.53	3765.54	1.41
2. Number of different funding sources	2.11	2.11	2.17	1.53	2.94	3.40**
3. Received special grants (first year)[a]	0.17	0.32	0.37	0.25	0.19	1.07
4. Received special grants (ever)[a]	0.29	0.36	0.40	0.41	0.44	0.34

[a] Coded as 0 = no, 1 = yes
** = $p < .01$.

retirement programs were the most likely to have been created for this purpose and senior citizens programs the least likely.

The 1984 per client budget ranged from $1,479.53 to $7,433.43. The more expensive models had more professional staff, had a larger number of staff, and operated on a full-time basis. There were significant differences among models in the number of different funding sources that contributed to their budgets, with leisure and outreach programs having the fewest sources and senior citizens programs the most. Less than one-third of the programs received special grants for the purpose of providing services to elderly mentally retarded persons during their first year of operation, and less than one-half received such grants at any point during their years of operation.

Program Characteristic Variables

Table 6-3 presents the results of a series of one-way analyses of variance in which the day program typology was the independent variable and program characteristics were the dependent variables.

As shown in Table 6-3, the day program models were significantly different with respect to the total number of clients served. The largest programs were the senior citizens programs; the smallest were leisure and outreach services. Although there were no significant differences among models in the number of elderly mentally retarded clients served, the types of programs did vary in the percentage of all clients who were elderly mentally retarded. In the four program models that primarily served mentally retarded clients, over three-fourths were elderly mentally retarded, while only one-fourth of all clients in the senior citizens programs surveyed were elderly mentally retarded.

The five types of day programs were also significantly different in the ratio of staff to clients. Day activity programs had the best ratio (1:4.95) while leisure and outreach services had the poorest (1:9.84).

At least two-thirds of the programs in each model provided their staff with special training on aging and retardation. Staff recommended that training be provided about generic services for the elderly and about the psychological aspects of aging. There were significant differences among the models with respect to the proportion of respondents who recommended that staff training be provided about the biological aspects of aging, with 100% of the vocational day programs making this recommendation as compared with only 25% of the senior citizens programs.

There were significant differences among the day program models with respect to the number of services provided to elderly mentally retarded clients. Specifically, models differed in their likelihood of providing medical, nursing, nutrition, psychological, social work, and self-care services. In general, leisure and outreach programs and supplemental retirement programs provided fewer types of formal services, while vocational day activity and senior citizens programs provided more.

More than 50% of the programs in each type used generic senior citizens services on behalf of their elderly mentally retarded clients. While, on the average, staff and clients from generic seniors programs were "somewhat receptive" to the participation of elderly mentally retarded clients, respondents indicated that staff in such programs were more receptive than were the clients.

Client Characteristic Variables

Table 6-4 presents the results of a series of one-way analyses of variance in which the day program typology was the independent variable

TABLE 6-3

Mean Values and Distributions for Program Characteristic Variables by Community Day Program Typology (N = 135)

VARIABLE	VOCA-TIONAL DAY ACTIVITY (n = 35)	DAY ACTIVITY (n = 37)	SUPPLE-MENTAL RETIRE-MENT (n = 30)	LEISURE AND OUTREACH (n = 17)	SENIOR CITIZENS CENTERS (n = 16)	F
A. *Size*						
1. Total number of clients	20.12	19.57	19.47	15.56	34.56	3.91**
2. Number of EMR clients	13.64	16.00	17.07	13.50	8.63	1.70
3. Percent EMR clients	76	88	88	88	26	38.07***
B. *Staffing*						
1. Total number of staff	4.56	5.08	2.79	3.06	5.41	2.11
2. Number of clients per one staff member	5.49	4.95	8.89	9.84	6.56	6.57***
3. Percent of programs with:						
a. Administrators	85	92	87	94	100	0.83
b. Nurses	41	53	10	6	73	9.03***
c. Therapists (OT, PT)	50	42	33	18	40	1.39
d. Psychologists	15	28	17	6	20	1.07
e. Social workers	41	44	37	29	47	0.37
f. Teachers	35	31	17	18	13	1.30
4. Percent programs providing staff training on aging	83	78	67	65	75	0.85
5. Percent programs recommending staff training on:						
a. Generic senior programs	50	25	30	33	0	0.71
b. Biological aspects of aging	100	50	90	50	25	3.23*
c. Psychological aspects of aging	50	38	60	50	25	0.40
C. *Services*						
1. Number of services to EMR clients	11.03	10.89	8.90	6.47	13.13	4.67***
2. Number of services to nonelderly MR clients	10.29	10.35	8.43	6.00	12.19	38.46**
3. Number of health services provided	1.43	1.41	0.57	0.24	1.75	6.61***
a. Percent providing medical	31	30	7	6	31	2.74*
b. Percent providing dental	17	11	3	0	6	1.53
c. Percent providing nursing	41	49	10	6	69	7.82***
d. Percent providing nutrition	56	51	37	12	69	3.81**

TABLE 6-3

Mean Values and Distributions for Program Characteristic Variables by Community Day Program Typology (N = 135) (Continued)

VARIABLE	VOCA-TIONAL DAY ACTIVITY (n = 35)	DAY ACTIVITY (n = 37)	SUPPLE-MENTAL RETIRE-MENT (n = 30)	LEISURE AND OUTREACH (n = 17)	SENIOR CITIZENS CENTERS (n = 16)	F
C. *Services* (Continued)						
4. Number of therapeutic services	1.86	1.76	1.33	0.88	2.38	2.95*
a. Percent providing PT or OT	49	41	33	24	63	1.71
b. Percent providing speech therapy	40	30	20	6	25	2.00
c. Percent providing psychological	43	43	27	12	56	2.51*
d. Percent providing social work	54	62	53	47	94	2.57*
5. Number of support services	1.17	1.27	1.17	0.94	1.50	1.05
a. Percent providing transportation	83	84	80	65	75	0.77
b. Percent providing financial assistance	17	27	23	29	50	1.60
c. Percent providing legal assistance	17	16	13	0	25	1.13
6. Number of educational services	1.54	1.35	1.30	1.12	1.75	2.46*
a. Percent providing adult education	60	46	50	47	75	1.21
b. Percent providing self-care	94	89	80	65	100	3.37**
7. Percent utilizing generic senior programs	63	73	77	50	100	3.10*
8. Senior centers staff receptivity rating[a]	2.59	2.42	2.36	2.88	2.43	1.39
9. Senior centers client receptivity rating[a]	2.43	2.19	2.14	2.13	2.13	0.65

[a] Rating scale: 1 = not at all receptive; 2 = somewhat receptive; 3 = very receptive
* = $p < .05$.　** = $p < .01$.　*** = $p < .001$

and client characteristics were the dependent variables. These data are descriptive of the elderly mentally retarded clients served in the five types of day programs.

As shown in Table 6-4, there were significant differences among the models with respect to the average age of clients, with vocational day activity programs having the youngest and senior citizens programs the oldest client groups. Notably, only about 10% of the clients served in the

TABLE 6-4

Distribution of Client Characteristic Variables by
Community Day Program Typology (N = 135)

VARIABLE[a]	VOCA-TIONAL DAY ACTIVITY (n = 35)	DAY ACTIVITY (n = 37)	SUPPLE-MENTAL RETIRE-MENT (n = 30)	LEISURE AND OUTREACH (n = 17)	SENIOR CITIZENS CENTERS (n = 16)	F
A. *Age*						
1. Average age (in age)	60.14	63.64	62.99	63.79	66.38	2.49*
2. Percent below age 22	0	0	0	0	0	—
3. Percent aged 22–50	13	8	6	7	11	0.90
4. Percent aged 51–54	13	6	6	7	4	2.34*
5. Percent aged 55–60	25	26	28	28	14	2.23
6. Percent aged 61–69	34	36	42	32	30	1.27
7. Percent aged 70 +	15	24	18	26	41	4.39**
8. Average age of:						
a. youngest client	46.20	48.69	50.37	49.29	47.38	0.61
b. oldest client	75.66	76.47	75.10	76.00	82.94	2.80*
B. *Gender*						
1. Percent female	47	61	57	55	65	2.63**
C. *Level of Retardation*						
1. Average level of MR[b]	0.84	0.91	1.10	1.27	1.26	3.62**
2. Percent mild	26	28	33	49	44	2.92*
3. Percent moderate	32	35	43	29	38	1.03
4. Percent severe or profound	42	37	24	22	18	3.24*
D. *Health*						
1. Average health ratings[c]	1.69	1.71	1.61	1.94	1.59	1.37
2. Percent in excellent health	12	16	11	21	7	0.80
3. Percent in good health	52	50	49	59	55	0.33
4. Percent in fair health	30	23	28	13	27	1.70
5. Percent in poor health	06	11	12	7	11	0.92
E. *Residential Placements*						
1. Percent in state schools	2	4	1	4	0	0.79
2. Percent in nursing homes	11	6	8	9	7	0.44
3. Percent in group homes	40	30	45	51	31	1.22
4. Percent in ICFs/MR	12	23	15	0	7	2.40*
5. Percent in apartment programs	1	4	4	2	7	0.49
6. Percent in foster homes	13	19	13	10	19	0.52
7. Percent with family	7	9	7	9	14	0.94
8. Percent in other placements	14	5	7	15	15	1.18

[a] The unit of analysis for variables in section A is the total client group in each program. The unit of analysis for variables in sections B through E is the elderly mentally retarded group in each program.   [b] Coded as: 2 = mild 1 = moderate 0 = severe or profound   [c] Coded as: 3 = excellent 2 = good 1 = fair 0 = poor per judgments of the respondents
* = $p < .05$.   ** = $p < .01$.

day program types were under the age of 50. While a larger proportion in all types of programs were age 70 or older, there were significant differences among models on this variable. Fully 41% of clients in senior citizens programs were age 70 or older while only 15% of those in vocational day activity programs were in this age category. The average age of the youngest client in these programs was in the late 40s, and the average age of the oldest client was in the late 70s or early 80s.

There were significant differences among models with respect to the proportion of males and females served. While only 47% of the clients in vocational day activity programs were female, two-thirds (65%) of those in senior citizens programs were female. This distribution of females versus males is correlated with the ages of clients in the various models. Program models with the oldest clients also had the highest percentage of females. The program types were also found to differ significantly in the level of retardation of clients. Vocational day activity programs served clients with the lowest cognitive skills, while leisure and outreach programs served clients with the highest cognitive skills. There were no significant differences among models in the reported health status of clients; more than 60% of the clients in each type were described as being in good or excellent health, given their age and disabilities.

About 10% of the clients who participated in the day program types lived in institutional settings (state schools and nursing homes). Just under 10% lived with their families. The modal residential placement of clients in each day program type was the group home. In general ICF/MR programs and foster homes were also frequently used placements. There were no significant between group differences in clients' residential placements, with the exception of ICF/MR placements, which were used by 23% of the clients in day activity programs and by none of the clients in leisure and outreach services.

CONCLUSIONS

Five distinct types of community-based day programs were identified from among the 135 programs that responded to the National Survey. Of the five types, senior citizens programs were the most unique in organizational context, program characteristics, and client characteristics, because they were a part of the aging services network.

The other four day program types were more centrally lodged within the mental retardation services network. As shown in Figure 6-1, a series of dimensions differentiates these four models in such a way that a continuum can be discerned among them: at one end is the vocational day activity program model, followed by day activity, then supplemental retirement, and finally leisure and outreach services at the other end.

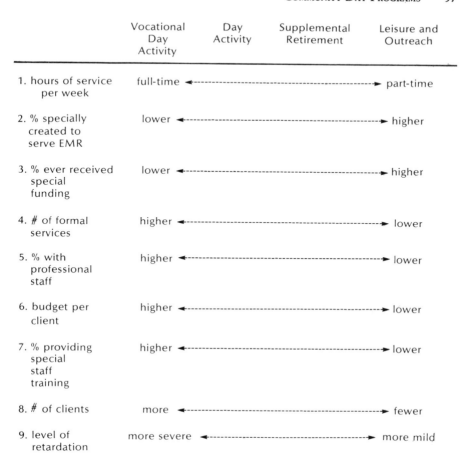

	Vocational Day Activity	Day Activity	Supplemental Retirement	Leisure and Outreach
1. hours of service per week	full-time ◄-	-	-	-► part-time
2. % specially created to serve EMR	lower ◄-	-	-	-► higher
3. % ever received special funding	lower ◄-	-	-	-► higher
4. # of formal services	higher ◄-	-	-	-► lower
5. % with professional staff	higher ◄-	-	-	-► lower
6. budget per client	higher ◄-	-	-	-► lower
7. % providing special staff training	higher ◄-	-	-	-► lower
8. # of clients	more ◄-	-	-	-► fewer
9. level of retardation	more severe ◄-	-	-	-► more mild

FIGURE 6-1: Dimensions Differentiating Four Day Program Models in the National Survey

Vocational day activity programs and, to a lesser extent, day activity programs tend to be modifications of existing models of day programs for younger retarded adults, while supplemental retirement programs and leisure and outreach services are newer innovations. Fewer of the first two types were created specifically for the purpose of providing services to elderly mentally retarded persons and a smaller proportion of these types received special funding. The first two types can be characterized as oriented more toward the provision of formal professionalized services, offering a greater number of professional services to clients, having a larger professional staff, and, as a consequence, having a higher per client budget. In contrast, supplemental retirement and leisure and outreach programs tend to be oriented more toward recreational activities than formal services.

The National Survey was not designed to collect outcome data about the effects of the different program models on the functional abilities or the quality of life of elderly mentally retarded persons. We also had no way in which to determine the relative effectiveness or appropriateness of the specialized day programs included in the National Survey as compared with traditional age-integrated day programs for mentally retarded adults. It is clear, however, from the findings presented in this chapter that there is a considerable amount of grassroots activity and that a range of innovative service options has been and is being developed.

Retirement options do exist. These will be explored at greater length in Chapter 10. Further, it is the norm for the day activity programs in the National Survey to utilize generic senior citizens services on behalf of their elderly mentally retarded clients, and there has been considerable success in doing so. The use of generic seniors programs will be examined in Chapter 9. The day programs surveyed have responded to the physical and mental limitations of the elderly clients they serve not by limiting their participation but rather by modifying the pacing of the day, developing new age-appropriate activities, and providing more support for them. These results are encouraging.

It should also be pointed out that the number of programs that exist and the number of clients served is small. The 135 day programs average out to 2 or 3 per state, although the pattern of distribution is in fact not even. In total they serve only about 2,000 elderly mentally retarded persons. In light of the excitement and interest of service providers in this population and the widely voiced belief that elderly mentally retarded persons are underserved, it is likely that the rate of program development will be very high in the next few years. Prospective studies in which the differential effects of the various day program models are examined would be particularly valuable in guiding program development initiatives. The key question remains, "What is the best match between client characteristics and needs on the one hand, and day program goals and services on the other?"

Chapter 7
Institutionally Based Residential and Day Programs

This chapter describes the 202 institutionally based programs that participated in the National Survey. It begins with a discussion of recent demographic shifts in the institutionalized population in this country and a review of the results of other studies regarding characteristics of institutionalized elderly mentally retarded persons. Detailed descriptions of the 140 institutionally based residential and 62 day programs primarily serving persons age 55 and over are then presented.

BACKGROUND

The population currently served in public residential facilities (institutions) is considerably older than the population served in the past. While in 1964–65, 49% of the residents of public institutions were aged 22 or older, by 1984–85 fully 83% were in this age group (Scheerenberger 1979; 1986). A series of interrelated trends is responsible for this change.

First, the proportion of children and youth residing in institutional facilities has decreased dramatically in recent years because very few young people have been admitted to such facilities and because there have been high rates of community placement of young institutional residents (Best-Sigford et al., 1982). The net effect is that the average age of those who remain in institutions has increased.

Second, disproportionately high rates of new admissions and re-admissions to public institutions occur among middle aged and elderly mentally retarded persons (Lakin, Hill, Hauber, Bruininks, & Heal, 1983). One reason for the increased rate of placement at these stages is related to the diminishing availability of family supports (Seltzer, 1985). As relatives age and are less able to care for an also aging mentally retarded family member, the probability of an out-of-home placement, particularly an institutional placement, increases substantially (Tausig, 1985). In their analysis of age-related placement patterns in New York state, Janicki and Jacobson (1986a) noted that "as they age, older developmentally disabled persons are less apt to live alone or with family and are more apt to live in institutions or in foster care" (p. 7). Similar findings have been reported by Meyers et al. (1985) for the state of California.

Third, residents of public institutions are "aging in place." The average life expectancy for mentally retarded persons has increased considerably during this century because of improved medical care (Eyman, Grossman, Tarjan, & Miller, 1987). The lower death rate of residents of public institutions further contributes to the increased proportion of elderly residents in such facilities.

Janicki and Jacobson's (1986a) New York state analysis, which provides a good indicator of national patterns, suggested that in the very near future elderly residents will comprise the majority of the population of many institutions. If the three trends noted above continue (i.e., if the placement of children in public institutions remains infrequent; if newly admitted clients tend to be middle aged or elderly; and if the average lifespan for mentally retarded persons stabilizes or continues to increase), a dominant client characteristic of residents of public institutions will be old age.

In order to plan programs and services for this aging institutional population, a series of key questions should be addressed. First, it is necessary to examine the characteristics of these elderly residents and to determine the extent to which they differ from two reference groups: younger institutionally based residents and elderly mentally retarded persons who reside in the community. Such comparisons will enable planners to assess the extent to which program models developed for these two reference groups are appropriate for elderly mentally retarded individuals.

A limited amount of past research is available in which comparisons are reported between older and younger institutionally based residents. Krauss and Seltzer (1986) compared four groups: those aged 22 to 54 and those aged 55 and older who lived in institutional and community settings in Massachusetts. As noted above in Chapter 2, when younger and older institutional residents were compared, the older residents were found to function at a higher level than did the younger residents. These data suggest that older institutionally based residents should not be excluded from day or residential programs on the basis of their age alone, as they seem to function at a higher level than do their younger counterparts. If special retirement programs are to be developed for aging institutionally based residents, these programs should be predicated not on the assumption of inferior functional skills, but rather on the possibility of expanded age-appropriate leisure activities.

Regarding the comparison of institutionally versus community-based elders, Krauss and Seltzer (1986) found that the institutionally based older subjects functioned at a lower level and had a greater number of impairments than did elderly residents in community settings. Janicki and Jacobson (1986b), in a cross-sectional analysis of generational trends in sensory, physical, and behavioral abilities of aging mentally retarded persons, reported a greater degree of age-related functional decline among institutionally based subjects than among community-based subjects. Similarly, Eyman and Arndt (1982) found that in California the older institutionally based subjects showed a decline in functional level in adulthood while those in the community continued to increase their skills.

These few studies suggest that service models developed for community-based elderly mentally retarded persons, such as those described in Chapters 5 and 6, may not necessarily be appropriate for the elderly residents of public institutions who are comparatively lower functioning.

A related question that should be examined by planners of institutional services for aging mentally retarded persons pertains to the extent to which the service needs of this population are met by the current range of services provided to them in public institutions. One key need is for an active day program. In their national probability sample, White et al., (1984) examined the availability of day placements for older institutionalized persons. They reported that with advancing age a higher number of clients have no day placement. Specifically, while only one-quarter (27.8%) of institutionalized adults aged 18 to 49 had no day placement, this was characteristic of nearly one-half (48.6%) of those aged 50 to 64 and nearly two-thirds (61.0%) of those over the age of 65. Having no formal day placement is particularly problematic for residents of public institutions because few alternative activities are available because of the geographic isolation of the facilities. Thus, service planners should consider the range of active retirement options that can be developed for elderly residents of institutions in order to respond to their diminished participation in traditional age-integrated day services.

THE NATIONAL SURVEY

The trends and issues discussed in the literature suggest that a steadily larger percentage of the institutionalized population can be classified as elderly. Consequently, institutions may well be one service sector in which innovative programming for elderly mentally retarded persons can be anticipated. One of the goals of the National Survey was to identify early attempts by public institutions to provide specialized day and residential services to this group. It was our expectation that as heterogeneous a set of programs would be identified in public institutions as had been located in community settings. In fact, while our analyses of both community residential and community day programs each generated a series of discrete types, we found that no comparable typologies emerged from the institutionally based programs surveyed. Instead, there was a remarkable degree of homogeneity within both residential and day institutionally based programs. This homogeneity may be in part a function of the influence of the ICF/MR status of many public institutions and the uniform requirements for active treatment, staffing, and physical facilities imposed by the ICF/MR regulations.

The remainder of this chapter presents detailed descriptions of institutionally based day and residential programs. Sixty-six public residential facilities or institutions located in 29 states participated in the National Survey. Institutions were included if they had a residential and/or a day program meeting the study's criteria (see Chapter 3). Of these 66 institutions, 29 (44%) had only residential programs, 28 (42%) had both residential and day programs, and 9 (14%) had only day programs for elderly mentally retarded persons.

In addition to the quantitative and qualitative descriptions, comparisons are made between the day and residential programs in order to explore how these different program functions are implemented for elderly mentally retarded persons. Prior to the discussion of these comparisons, two case studies are presented in order to highlight the qualitative dimensions of institutionally based programs.

CASE EXAMPLES

Institutionally Based Residential Program

The Adult Care Services Unit, which is located in a midwestern public institution, served 64 older mentally retarded persons in four 16-bed cottages. The cottages were constructed in 1982. At that time, the institution made a philosophical change in programming for elderly mentally retarded persons. According to the Unit's director, prior to 1982, "it had been the basic stance that individual clients were assessed and programs designed to develop self-help skills. Always the goal was toward more independence. . . . However, as clients aged, it became necessary to re-assess their needs. We found, for example, that there were clients in the institution who probably would never be placed in the community. Therefore, their aging process should be recognized and planned for accordingly."

Each of the four cottages contained eight bedrooms with two clients in each room, a day room measuring 15' × 15', and two bathrooms. Meals were served elsewhere in the institution. The four cottages shared a common outdoor courtyard. Institution vehicles were assigned to this program, and seemed to satisfy the transportation needs of the four cottages. Two of the cottages served male clients and two served female clients.

Although the minimum age for admission was 55 years, exceptions have been made for younger adults who have "plateaued in their development of new skills and whose health has deteriorated." Each cottage had clients in their 50s, 60s, and 70s. Over three-quarters (76.5%) of the 64 clients were severely or profoundly retarded. In two of the cottages (one serving men and one women) clients were all classified as being in fair or poor health, while in the other two cottages, nearly all of the clients were in good or excellent health.

The director of the unit explained that "the emphasis in programming becomes one of retaining previously developed skills as long as possible. Their schedule shifts to leisure activities, including arts and crafts, recreation, participation in community activities, and participation in social activities in the cottage." Each of the four cottages had made a different set of arrangements to implement this programming emphasis. All female clients participated in formal day programs held in the two cottages in which they lived. One of the cottages for males sent all of them to an on-grounds age-integrated day activity center, while the other sent half of its clients to the day activity center and the other half to an on-grounds recreational program.

There was an increasing demand for admission to the Adult Care Services Unit both from long term institutionalized clients who have reached old age and from elderly clients recently placed in the institution after their community-based placements were no longer able to maintain them. The long term potential of this unit was best expressed by the staff member who noted, "While our clients may not be able to learn to independently purchase coffee in a cafe, we can let them participate in this activity for its sheer enjoyment potential."

Institutionally Based Day Program

The Geriatrics Life Activities Program is located in a public residential facility in a northeastern state. It operated from 8:30 to 11:30 AM and from 1:00 to 2:30 PM five days a week. According to the program's director, the Geriatric Life Activities Program was established in 1980 to offer services and activities to a wide range of aging clients. Special emphasis was placed on maintaining previously acquired skills while increasing social awareness and life skills.

The program served 21 clients at the time of the survey, all but one of whom were over the age of 55. The youngest client was 52 years of age and had Down syndrome and Alzheimer's disease. The remaining clients ranged from 55 to 80 years of age. The director reported that 19 of the 20 elderly clients were severely or profoundly retarded and had substantial secondary disabilities and handicapping conditions such as cerebral palsy, epilepsy, visual and hearing impairments, arthritis, and stroke. In spite of these chronic conditions, 15 clients were reported to be in good or excellent health. All lived in an age-integrated residential unit on the grounds of the institution.

Clients were referred to the program by an interdisciplinary team that assessed whether an older individual was in need of a retirement program. Age alone was not the basis for a referral. A client must also have had a loss of skills and a reduced motivation for participating in an age-integrated day program.

The Geriatric Life Activities Program was staffed by one full-time administrator (who founded the program), 1.5 direct care staff members who accompanied the clients from the residence and who assisted the administrator, and consulting occupational, physical, and recreational therapists, psychologists, social workers, and chaplains.

The physical setting occupied by the program was a large ground floor room that had been partitioned into three areas: a living area with lounge chairs, a couch, and a stereo system; a fine motor/sensory stimulation area; and an area with tables and chairs that was set up for tabletop activities and as a kitchen. Outside there was a lawn with outdoor furniture and a garden. The director of the program explained that the staff had worked hard to improve this space to meet the needs of the clients. They successfully advocated for the addition of a back door to make the space accessible to clients in wheelchairs, added brighter lighting for visually impaired clients, and were in the process of recovering all of the tabletops with black contact paper in order to enable clients to make finer figure-ground discriminations. This program has operated since its inception without any special grants.

The clients who participated in the Geriatric Life Activities Program engaged in the following activities every week: bowling, cooking, swimming, music, exercise class, and a community trip. These activities were generally scheduled for the mornings, while in the afternoons staff worked with clients on an individual or small group basis. To respond to the special needs posed by their elderly clients, staff tended to schedule activities for shorter periods of time, provided frequent opportunities for rest, and were cautious about the client's health. The program routinely used institution vehicles for transportation and the director reported that their transportation needs were fully met.

The Geriatrics Life Activities Program had an active volunteer program. Retired citizens from the local community organized the clients as a chapter of the RSVP (Retired Senior Volunteer Program). In this way the Geriatric Life Activities clients engaged in volunteer activities on behalf of other clients in the institution, such as making holiday decorations for other units, making Valentine cards, and baking birthday cakes.

The program currently has a long waiting list. To respond to the increasing need for special services for the institution's growing aging population, plans have been made to relocate the Geriatrics Life Activities Program to a larger space connected to a specialized residential unit for elderly mentally retarded persons.

Summary

The qualitative descriptions of institutionally based residential and day programs reveal the various ways in which the needs of elderly mentally retarded clients are reflected in the purpose, structure, and content of the programs. The remainder of this chapter presents more detailed information on these areas through quantitative descriptions of these two program components of public institutions.

PROGRAM ORIENTATION
HISTORY

Overview of Program Goals

Respondents were asked to describe the goals of the residential or day program included in the National Survey. A sample of their responses is presented in Table 7-1. Common themes evident in the descriptions for residential programs include the emphasis on maintaining clients' current skill levels, developing leisure interests, and attending to health and medical needs. Respondents clearly contrasted these emphases with other institutional programs in which skill building and growth are espoused.

Respondents for institutionally based day programs typically described the wide variety of recreational activities provided in the programs. Many noted that the schedule or pace of events had been modified in deference to clients' reduced energy levels.

Program Development History

Institutionally based residential programs were slightly older than institutionally based day programs. The average year in which residential programs opened was 1980 as compared with 1982 for day programs. Further, 1982 was the year in which the largest number of institutionally based residential programs were opened, while for day programs 1984 was the modal year of opening. Given that the survey was conducted in 1985, it is notable that many of the programs included were of very recent origin.

Almost three-quarters (72.6%) of the institutionally based day pro-

TABLE 7-1

Selected Descriptions of Institutionally Based Residential and Day Program Goals

Residential Programs
- Our unit is part of a community living skills unit. We were originally a geriatric unit but we are now serving clients who also have ambulation problems. We try to keep clients active but we are not now focused on community living skills.
- The cottage, one of 13 at the institution, is designated to serve older residents who need a less strenuous environment. We try to maintain the residents' current level of functioning and to protect them from more aggressive younger residents. We are not trying to place these residents in the community.
- This residential program is for six clients who also receive feeding, positioning, and educational day programs. The unit offers active, modified recreational programs including field trips. Our goal is to maintain clients' current functioning, not to provide active treatment.
- The program provides the institutionalized aged with a nonstrenuous learning environment within which to maintain skills, develop new interests, participate in meaningful activities, and enjoy retirement. The program serves 75 clients aged 52–97 with a full range of functional levels and needs.
- This program is for the highest functioning of our geriatric population. We have no dual diagnosis or behavior problems clients. Some work on grounds and are paid through the sheltered workshop. In the afternoon, they go to a retirement center. Within the residential unit, they have access to board games, foster grandparents program and a strong emphasis on leisure/socialization.
- This program is for the more medically involved. Fifteen are in wheelchairs. Our main focus is on maintaining health and functional skills. Six clients are both mentally retarded and mentally ill and are monitored by psychiatrists.
- The cottage is a residence for 20 women all over 40 years of age. We are more progressive in geriatric treatment than the other cottages. The program's goal is to make clients as comfortable as possible and give clients more choices and independence than younger clients have.
- The program is one of four apartment units in the infirmary. Most residents have severe medical needs and get 24-hour nursing care from the residence staff. Our programming is aimed toward maintaining health and functional level.
- The cottage is not set up differently from other cottages except that the pace is more leisurely. Thirty-nine of the clients are over 55 years old. The specialists (such as the physical therapist, occupational therapist, and psychologist) come to the cottage instead of the clients going to them.

Day Programs
- Our clients are involved in two types of activities: social groups, where we have discussions based on what the clients want to talk about; and crafts, where we teach people hobbies such as cooking. We can sell their crafts at a bazaar held on the grounds.
- The focus is on maintenance of skills, on leisure or recreational skills and on creative expression. The program is individualized and stresses image-enhancing activities and age-appropriate activities.
- Clients spend 3 hours in the morning and 2 hours in the afternoon at the program. Each client has activity goals such as leather work, quilting, etc. They can sell their crafts at our Christmas Fair. We also provide social and recreational activities such as trips to see movies.
- The program was developed to serve clients who physically could not participate in regular programs. The program has a library, arts and crafts, domestic skills, moderate exercises, outings, and horticulture. We serve two groups of clients for 4 hours a day for each group.

TABLE 7-1

Selected Descriptions of Institutionally Based Residential and Day Program Goals (Continued)

- The program lasts 6 hours a day because of the requirements of the regulations. We begin with reality orientation, nature appreciation (feeding fish, watering plants), discuss death and dying, and have pets brought in once a month. Refreshments are served. We also have "down" time for relaxation, arts and crafts, and music.
- This day program is for elderly clients who are able to leave the residential area. We try to meet the special needs of elderly institutional clients who are not well served by vocational programs. The program tries to allow retirement type opportunities. We also provide ADL skills, OT, PT, etc., as needed. We have three groups. The lowest functioning get ADL skills; the moderate functioning have a recreational focus; the highest functioning group is preparing for community placement.

grams, versus slightly less than half (49.3%) of the residential programs, were specifically created to serve elderly persons ($\chi^2 = 8.56$, $p < .01$). This difference between residential and day programs parallels the findings presented in Chapters 5 and 6 in which the community-based residential programs were generally adaptations of pre-existing models, while community-based day programs were more often new program types.

Respondents described a variety of motivations or reasons for the program's initiation. For example, one noted that "these people were just lying in bed and being turned over by nurses so we felt a program was needed." Another said that "a decision was made to serve clients with high medical risks." Many others stated that the programs were started to serve clients whose ambulation or health status made continued participation in traditional programs difficult.

Program Entrance Criteria

Most of the residential (97.1%) and day programs (95.2%) had at least one entrance criterion. While these criteria were not always strictly applied, respondents indicated that either formally or informally the criteria were used to select program participants. As shown in Table 7-2, significant differences between day and residential programs were found for only three entrance criteria: age, functional skills, and medical status. Age was a selection criterion in virtually all residential programs but only in three-quarters of the day programs. Functional skills were also more likely to be used by residential programs than day programs in selecting clients. In contrast, day programs were more likely than residential programs to have medical status criteria as a basis for client selection.

About two-thirds (69.5%) of the day programs and slightly more than

TABLE 7-2

Criteria Used for Client Selection in Institutionally Based
Residential and Day Programs

CRITERION	RESIDENTIAL ($n = 140$)	DAY ($n = 62$)	t
Age	90.7%	75.8%	2.48*
Functional skills	62.1	45.2	2.27*
Sensory impairments	28.6	32.3	−.53
Medical status	19.3	35.5	−2.50**
Pre-existing social groups	2.1	8.1	−1.60
Behavior problems	4.3	1.6	1.13
Gender	5.0	0.0	1.80

$* = p<.05.$ $** = p<.01.$

half (56.6%) of the residential programs specified a minimum age limit for program participation. The most commonly used minimum age limit was 55 years (for 39.7% of residential and 82.9% of day programs that had minimum age requirements).

Program Size

Residential programs were significantly smaller in size than day programs (mean = 25.9 and 35.2, respectively, $t = -2.38$, $p < .05$). The range in size for both residential and day programs, however, was very broad. For residential programs, the modal number of clients was 8 while the range was 6 to 100 residents. For day programs, the modal number of participants was 11 and the range in size was 4 to 176.

CLIENT CHARACTERISTICS

Information was collected on the age, sex, level of mental retardation, presence of additional disabilities, and health status of the participants in the institutionally based residential and day programs.

Age

Clients served in institutionally based day programs were significantly older (mean = 63.95) than clients served in institutionally based residential programs (mean = 61.81, $t = -2.33$, $p < .05$). Table 7-3 illustrates the considerable variability between residential and day programs in the percentage of participants in different age categories.

Consistent with these programs' focus on providing services to elderly clients, no day program and only two residential programs served anyone

TABLE 7-3

Percentage of Clients in Institutionally Based Residential and Day Programs by Age Category

AGE CATEGORY	RESIDENTIAL (n = 140)	DAY (n = 62)	t
Less than 22 yrs	0.1%	0.0%	.34
22–50 years	15.1	7.8	3.64***
51–54 years	7.5	7.3	.23
55–60 years	19.2	22.0	−1.25
61–69 years	33.3	37.7	−1.87
70+ years	24.8	25.2	−.11

*** = $p < .001$.

under 22 years of age. Fully half of the day programs (45.9%) and about a quarter (26.7%) of the residential programs served no one under 51 years of age. On average, a significantly greater percentage of the clients in day programs (85%) than residential programs (78%) were age 55 or over ($t = -2.81$, $p < .01$).

Sex

There were more females than males among the elderly participants in residential and day programs (57.2% and 51.4%, respectively). Over half (59.3%) of the residential programs served only males or females, while virtually all the day programs were sex integrated (see Table 7-4).

Level of Retardation

Table 7-5 presents data on percentage of program participants over age 55 by level of retardation for residential and day programs. These clients were largely severely or profoundly retarded (68.1% of residential and 72.6% of day programs). Indeed, 18.6% of the residential programs and 21% of the day programs served only severely or profoundly retarded persons.

TABLE 7-4

Percentage of Sex Segregated Institutionally Based Residential and Day Programs

PROGRAM TYPE	RESIDENTIAL (n = 140)	DAY (n = 62)	t
All male program	22.9%	3.2%	4.65***
All female program	36.4	6.5	5.82***
Sex integrated	40.7	90.3	−8.81***

*** = $p < .001$.

TABLE 7-5

Percentage of Elderly Mentally Retarded Clients by Level of Retardation and Type of Institutionally Based Programs

LEVEL OF RETARDATION	RESIDENTIAL (n = 140)	DAY (n = 62)	t
Mild	14.7%	10.7%	1.63
Moderate	17.2	16.6	.21
Severe	37.5	35.4	.57
Profound	30.6	37.3	−1.43

Additional Disabilities

All residential and day programs served elderly clients who had disabilities in addition to their retardation. The percentages of program participants with various types of disabilities are shown in Table 7-6. These data reveal considerable similarity between day program and residential program clients in their additional disabilities in spite of the age difference between these two groups of clients. Very few residential programs had a resident with an additional disability of autism (only five programs) or Alzheimer's disease (21 programs). Only eight residential programs served residents who had both Down syndrome and Alzheimer's disease.

Almost all (91.2%) of the participants in residential programs were described as being incapable of self-preservation (i.e., unable to independently evacuate a building within 2 ½ minutes).

TABLE 7-6

Percentage of Elderly Mentally Retarded Participants in Institutionally Based Residential and Day Programs with Various Additional Disabilities[a]

DISABILITY	RESIDENTIAL (n = 140)	DAY (n = 62)	t
Epilepsy	21.9%	20.1%	.50
Nonverbal	21.1	29.6	−2.34*
Nonambulatory	18.0	17.9	.03
Emotional problems	11.4	10.2	.50
Visual impairments	20.4	26.4	.76
Hearing impairments	22.2	21.2	.32
Cerebral palsy	3.7	5.4	−1.08
Autism	.6	.2	.93
Alzheimer's Disease	1.8	3.8	−1.01
Down syndrome	5.4	7.4	−1.14

[a] Percentages do not add to 100% because individuals can have multiple disabilities.
* = $p < .05$.

Health Status

Respondents were asked to characterize the health status of participants who were over age 55 as either excellent, good, fair, or poor given the individual's age and level of disability. The majority of participants in institutionally based residential and day programs were rated as being in either good or excellent health (54.1% and 55.7%, respectively). Only 14.2% of clients in day programs and 10.3% of those in residential programs were said to be in poor health.

PROGRAM CHARACTERISTICS

Physical Location

Two-thirds (65.5%) of the residential programs occupied an entire building on the institution grounds, while almost a third (30.2%) shared the building with other residential units. The other six residential programs were located in off-grounds buildings. In contrast, most of the day programs (86.2%) occupied part of a building on the institution grounds and only 12.0% occupied an entire building. The one remaining day program was located in a building off the institution grounds.

Almost two-thirds of the sites for both residential programs (62.3%) and day programs (61.3%) had been physically renovated during the previous decade. An additional third (31.2%) of the residential programs and a fifth (21.0%) of the day programs were described as located on newly constructed sites, leaving only 6.5% of the residential programs and 17.7% of the day program operating in unrenovated older facilities.

Physical and Social Integration of Day Programs

Respondents from institutionally based day programs were asked to describe the extent to which their elderly program participants were physically and socially integrated with younger mentally retarded participants (see Table 7-7). Less than a quarter of the programs described their elderly participants as fully integrated (either physically or socially) with their younger participants. This may reflect the large percentage (72.6%) of institutionally based day programs that were specially created to serve the elderly group and the fact that nearly one-fifth (19.4%) of the institutionally based programs did not serve persons younger than age 55.

It is interesting to note that physical and social integration seemed to go hand in hand. However, as noted earlier, many respondents stated that their programs were designed to provide an alternative to integrated

TABLE 7-7

Physical and Social Integration of Elderly Mentally Retarded Persons in Institutionally Based Day Programs ($N = 62$)

DEGREE OF INTEGRATION	PHYSICAL INTEGRATION	SOCIAL INTEGRATION
Not integrated	40.3%	39.3%
Sometimes integrated	37.1	41.0
Always integrated	22.6	19.7

programs including younger mentally retarded persons. Thus, the high degree of segregation of these programs was not surprising.

Hours of Operation of Day Programs

The 62 day programs were asked to describe their hours of operation. While the mean number of hours per week that day programs were open was 30 hours, there was a range of between 3 and 75 hours per week. Over two-thirds (69.4%) operated five days a week for at least 6 hours per day. Most of the other programs were open five days a week for less than 6 hours a day (18 or 29% of the day programs). One program was in operation only during the evening and weekend hours.

Program Activities: Day Programs

Respondents were asked about the frequency with which different types of activities were offered within the programs to their elderly participants. These activities were categorized into five general types: activities of daily living, academic/vocational, social and interpersonal skills, health, and leisure activities (see Table 7-8).

About half of the day programs provided personal hygiene, grooming, and eating skills training on a daily basis. Very few programs offered academic or vocational components. Training for community integration, including money identification and travel training, were never provided by 62% and 59% of the programs, respectively. When offered, they were likely to be provided on a weekly basis.

Social and interpersonal skills training presented a more mixed pattern. While few programs said they had behavior management components (over half never provided it), the majority of the day programs said they provided social skills training and reality orientation on a daily basis. Communication skills training was typically provided on either a weekly or daily basis.

With respect to the two health related activities, exercise programs

TABLE 7-8

Activities in Institutionally Based Day Programs (N = 62)

	NEVER	FREQUENCY OF PROVISION AT LEAST MONTHLY	AT LEAST WEEKLY	DAILY
Activities of daily living				
Personal hygiene	33.9%	8.1%	3.2%	54.8%
Personal grooming	25.8	11.3	12.9	50.0
Feeding/eating	40.3	8.1	3.2	48.4
Academic/Vocational				
Academic skills	75.4	6.6	11.5	6.5
Vocational	86.9	13.1	0.0	0.0
Pre-vocational	62.9	37.1	0.0	0.0
Money identification and handling	62.3	9.8	21.3	6.6
Travel training	59.0	16.4	21.3	3.3
Social and interpersonal skills				
Social skills	4.8	8.1	19.4	67.7
Reality orientation	22.6	3.2	16.1	58.1
Behavior management	54.8	16.2	11.3	17.7
Communication skills	27.4	9.7	30.6	32.3
Health				
Nutritional education	71.0	6.4	11.3	11.3
Exercise programs	22.6	4.8	27.4	45.2
Leisure activities				
Community trips	14.8	36.1	45.9	3.2
Gardening	46.8	14.5	24.2	14.5
Arts and crafts	6.5	9.7	38.7	45.1
Organized games	35.5	11.3	38.7	14.5
Movies	32.3	33.9	30.6	3.2
Music	19.3	6.5	45.2	29.0
Religious services	74.2	8.1	16.1	1.6
Sports programs	53.2	8.1	33.9	4.8

were provided by almost half the programs on a daily basis. Over two-thirds of the day programs did not provide any nutritional education to their elderly participants.

A variety of leisure activities were provided by day programs. Over half of the programs reported that they scheduled community trips, organized games and/or sports, and offered musical activities, most commonly on a weekly basis. Arts and crafts were offered by virtually all of the programs, most commonly on a daily basis. Few day programs included religious components.

Program Activities: Residential Programs

Comparable information on the range and frequency of provision of activities within residential programs is presented in Table 7-9. All three

TABLE 7-9

Activities in Institutionally Based Residential Programs (N = 140)

	NEVER	FREQUENCY OF PROVISION AT LEAST MONTHLY	AT LEAST WEEKLY	DAILY
Activities of daily living				
Personal hygiene	7.1%	.8%	1.4%	90.7%
Personal grooming	8.6	.7	2.8	87.9
Feeding/eating	29.3	2.1	3.6	65.0
Academic/Vocational				
Academic skills	79.3	2.9	12.1	5.7
Vocational	87.8	12.2	0.0	0.0
Pre-vocational	77.9	22.1	0.0	0.0
Money identification and handling	73.4	7.2	14.4	5.0
Travel training	87.8	5.8	4.3	2.1
Social and interpersonal skills				
Social skills	25.7	5.0	15.0	54.3
Reality orientation	46.8	11.5	24.5	17.2
Behavior management	65.7	5.8	3.6	24.9
Communication skills	55.0	6.4	25.7	12.9
Health				
Nutritional education	76.4	5.7	7.2	10.7
Exercise programs	42.9	2.8	35.0	19.3
Leisure activities				
Community trips	12.9	31.7	54.7	.7
Gardening	79.3	5.7	11.4	3.6
Arts and crafts	21.4	10.0	50.7	17.9
Organized games	25.7	10.0	54.3	10.0
Movies	10.7	15.7	72.9	.7
Music	30.2	19.4	29.5	20.9
Religious services	14.3	5.0	80.7	0.0
Sports programs	59.4	12.1	27.1	1.4

activities of daily living were provided by the vast majority of residential programs on a daily basis.

Very few residential programs offered academic or vocational skills development components within their programs.

Social and interpersonal skills training were provided on a more variable basis than was found for day programs. While social skills training was provided by over half of the residential programs on a daily basis, less than half of the programs provided either behavior management or communication skills training.

Although over half of the residential programs provided exercise programs on either a weekly or daily basis, few provided nutritional education for their elderly residents.

Leisure activities, when provided, were commonly offered on a weekly basis. The most frequently provided activities were community trips and movies (by almost 90%). Arts and crafts, organized games, and religious services were also commonly offered on a weekly basis. The majority of residential programs also offered musical activities, although the frequency varied considerably.

Program Activities: Comparison Between Residential and Day Programs

Table 7-10 presents a more direct comparison of the frequency with which various types of activities were provided by residential and day programs. Residential programs provided training in activities for daily living significantly more frequently than did day programs. There was

TABLE 7-10

Comparison of the Average Frequency[a] of Service Provision Between Institutionally Based Residential and Day Programs

	RESIDENTIAL (n = 140)	DAY (n = 62)	t
Activities of daily living			
Personal hygiene	2.76	1.79	5.07***
Personal grooming	2.70	1.87	4.63***
Feeding/eating	2.04	1.59	2.11*
Academic/Vocational			
Academic skills	.44	.49	−.35
Vocational	.12	.13	−.17
Pre-vocational	.22	.37	−2.23
Money identification and handling	.51	.72	−1.44
Travel training	.21	.69	−3.71***
Social and interpersonal skills			
Social skills	1.98	2.50	−3.43***
Reality orientation	1.12	2.10	−5.32***
Behavior management	.88	.92	−.22
Communication skills	.96	1.68	−4.01***
Health			
Nutritional education	.52	.63	−.68
Exercise programs	1.31	1.95	−3.52***
Leisure activities			
Community trips	1.43	1.38	.48
Gardening	.39	1.06	−4.71***
Arts and crafts	1.65	2.23	−3.89***
Organized games	1.49	1.32	1.04
Movies	1.64	1.05	4.69***
Music	1.41	1.84	−2.60**
Religious services	1.66	.45	10.04***
Sports programs	.71	.90	−1.35

[a] Coded as 0 = never, 1 = at least monthly, 2 = at least weekly, 3 = daily
$* = p<.05.$ $** = p<.01.$ $*** = p<.001.$

only one type of academic/vocational activity in which there was a significant difference between residential and day programs: travel training. The low mean frequency scores for the five activities in this category suggests that these activities are of only minor importance to institutionally based residential and day programs.

Day programs were significantly more likely to provide more frequent training in three of the four activities in the social and interpersonal skills category and in one of the two health-related activities. Significant differences were found with respect to the frequency with which leisure activities were provided in day and residential programs. Day programs provided gardening, arts and crafts, and music programs more regularly than did residential programs. Residential programs provided movies and religious programs more regularly than did day programs.

Staffing of Programs

The average number of clients per staff member was 1.1 for institutionally based residential programs, versus an average of 5.9 clients per staff for day programs. The difference was statistically significant ($t = -5.7, p < .001$).

In order to compare the types of staff employed in residential and day programs, the percentage of programs that had at least .1 FTE (full-time equivalent) for various types of staff was calculated (see Table 7-11). As expected, virtually all the programs had administrators and direct care staff. Significant differences were found between residential and day programs with respect to almost all other types of staff employed. Over

TABLE 7-11

Percentage of Institutionally Based Residential and Day Programs Having at Least .1 FTE of Staff

TYPE OF STAFF	RESIDENTIAL (n = 140)	DAY (n = 62)	t
Administrators	100.0%	95.2%	1.50
Direct care staff	99.3	83.9	3.42***
Physicians	58.6	14.5	7.00***
Recreation staff	79.3	56.4	3.21**
Therapists	57.1	43.5	1.74
Psychologists	75.0	43.5	4.44***
Teachers	29.3	41.9	−16.15***
Nurses	95.7	37.1	9.30***
Social workers	81.4	25.8	8.83***
Other	37.9	21.0	2.38**

** $= p < .01$.   *** $= p < .001$.

three-quarters of the residential programs (79.3%) but only about half of the day programs (56.4%) employed recreational staff. Health professionals (i.e., physicians and nurses) were more commonly associated with residential than with day programs. In general, residential programs were more likely to have professional staff than were day programs.

In almost half (46%) of the residential programs, staff from the residence were also assigned to the day programs in which the elderly mentally retarded clients participated. The most frequently shared staff were as follows: direct care staff (78.8% of residential programs), recreational staff (57.6% of programs), psychologists (50%), therapists (43.9%), social workers (39.4%), nurses (30.3%), administrators (22.7%), teachers (19.7%), and physicians (10.6%).

The extent to which staff are trained to work with elderly mentally retarded persons is a recurrent issue in the literature. The data collected for the National Survey suggests that institutionally based staff who are assigned to programs serving elderly clients are provided with at least some specialized training. Fully 84% of the respondents for day programs and 74% of the respondents for residential programs reported that special training sessions had been offered to staff. The average number of hours of training during the preceding six months was 7.4 for staff in day programs and 5.1 for staff in residential programs. The most commonly provided type of training was in-service workshops (for 88% of the residential programs and 67% of the day programs). Other methods of training included outside seminars and distribution of written materials.

Respondents were asked to describe the types of information they thought were most valuable to staff. Information on the physical aspects of the aging process was most often identified as important (cited by 84% and 71% of the residential and day programs, respectively), followed by information on aging in general (cited by 78% and 68% of the programs, respectively). Other areas mentioned included information on the aging process for mentally retarded/developmentally disabled persons in particular, and on the emotional aspects of aging. Interestingly, only 23% of the respondents for residential programs (compared with 47% of the respondents for day programs) said that visiting other programs was an important training method for staff ($t = -3.27$, $p<.001$).

Day Program Placements of Clients in Residential Programs

Respondents from the residential programs were asked to identify the percentage of the residents in their units who participated in the same day program. In a quarter of the residential programs (25.2%), all of the elderly residents attended the same day program. Thus, for these clients, the people with whom they lived were also the people with whom they spent their days. For another quarter of the residential programs (23.0%), respondents said that between three-quarters and 99% of the elderly residents attended the same day program, while in an equal percentage of programs (23.0%) the respondents said that between half and three-quarters of the elderly residents attended the same day program. In summary, in almost three-quarters of the institutionally based residential programs, at least half of the elderly residents attended day programs together.

In 34 of the residential programs (24.5%), there was a retirement option for the residents, meaning that clients could elect to participate in a nontraditional day program, including staying within the residence during the day and/or attending recreational as opposed to vocationally oriented day programs. Appropriately, the client's preference was the primary basis for allowing residents to exercise the retirement option in 74% of these programs. Other bases included the client's medical status (cited by 62% of programs) and age or functional status (each cited by 29% of programs). Interestingly, the availability of daytime staff and/or the availability of alternative programs was cited as the basis for retirement decisions by respondents in only three programs. Thus, while the prevalence of retirement options was not widespread for the clients who lived in the residential programs surveyed, the bases on which this option was exercised related strongly to client rather than programmatic or staffing concerns.

Where do clients who have exercised a retirement option spend their days? In 14 programs, all of the retired clients stayed at the residence, with either no formal program (five programs), informal programs (eight programs), or a formal day program (one program). In the other programs, retired clients attended a special program on the grounds of the institution. In only one residential program were retired clients placed in a special program off the institution grounds.

SPECIAL CONCERNS
OF PROGRAMS

Residential and day program respondents were asked whether they faced any special concerns or issues in providing care for elderly mentally retarded persons (see Table 7-12). The most frequently mentioned issue for both residential and day programs was dealing with medically fragile clients (cited by over 80%). Programs reported a variety of strategies for approaching this issue. Some concentrated on augmenting staff skills by

TABLE 7-12

Special Issues Faced by Institutionally Based Residential and Day Programs in Serving Elderly Mentally Retarded Persons

TYPE OF ISSUE	RESIDENTIAL (n = 140)	DAY (n = 62)	t
Dealing with medically fragile clients	84.3%	87.1%	−.53
Providing retirement or alternate activities	80.7	51.6	1.23
Dealing with death and dying issues	78.6	66.1	1.79
Dealing with client's family	70.7	48.4	2.99**
Need for physical facility renovation	40.0	72.6	−1.52

** = p<.01.

providing training about age-related changes in clients' behavior or physical symptomology. Other programs noted that they relied on the institution's interdisciplinary teams and health care professionals to monitor health and behavioral changes. Another strategy was to develop closer linkages with community hospitals and physicians that provide outpatient care for some institutionally based clients.

Most institutions had an infirmary and many respondents reported that some of their clients had been placed in the infirmary for acute illnesses. It was noted earlier that almost all of the residential and over a third of the day programs had a nurse as part of the program's staff. However, respondents also noted either the existence of or the need for a skilled nursing care unit within the institution for clients who needed long term nursing services.

Some respondents noted that they tried to involve chronically ill clients in ongoing activities. One day program director said that staff "try to let clients participate as much as they feel comfortable. We also have other clients make cards for or visit ill clients." Another program respondent was frank about the impact on staff who "expect to see progress and have a hard time accepting that some clients can only be maintained at the current level of functioning. We're trying to get more LPNs (Licensed Practical Nurses) and nursing aide staff."

Another commonly cited issue for programs was providing retirement or alternative activities for residents. Many of the day programs surveyed described themselves as the institution's retirement option. However, some respondents expressed concern over the appropriateness of retirement for mentally retarded persons because they feared that retirement would mean withdrawal from active involvement in formal programs. Others noted that Medicaid regulations require clients to participate in "active treatment" programs for 6 hours per day. These regulations were described as curbing the extent to which programmatic changes are possible to allow clients more relaxed or flexible schedules.

Helping clients cope with the death of family members or friends was another concern for programs. Many respondents said that the social work departments in the institutions had primary responsibility for formal activities in this area. Social workers provided individual counseling for clients and in some cases established support groups for clients, staff, or both together. Other respondents noted that in-service training was provided to staff in their programs to help them learn effective ways of assisting clients during bereavement. One program said that after a client had died, a memorial service was held in which the other clients participated.

The involvement of program staff with clients' families was another issue frequently mentioned by respondents, although cited more often by residential program staff than by day program respondents. Program involvement with immediate and extended family members varied from little or no contact (because the family members were themselves old or deceased or because thy had lost touch after many decades of their family member's institutionalization), to informal contact around social events and holidays, to formal contact (through family members' participation in program planning activities). Many respondents stated that they encouraged family visits and that correspondence was sent at least quarterly. However, one respondent's comments echoed those of many. "Almost all our clients have no family ties. We're their family. Really, their relationships are with paid staff."

Providing a physical environment that supports clients' needs is obviously another important issue for programs. Many respondents noted that physical renovations had either been completed or were in the planning/discussion stage. Typical renovations included making the program area accessible to wheelchairs, placing grab-bars in bathrooms and handrails in the hallways, and increasing the lighting. Most programs that had not had renovations said that they have requested physical modifications but were realistically expecting considerable delay before completion.

Programs were also asked if they perceived the needs of elderly clients as being different from those of younger mentally retarded persons (see Table 7-13). For both residential and day programs, the most frequently cited difference was with respect to clients' physical health care needs. For example, respondents noted these clients needed more exercise and physical care and less active programs because of increasing frailty. Roughly two-thirds of the programs, irrespective of type, noted that elderly mentally retarded persons had special needs with respect to the types of services they required, the activities they preferred and the energy levels they could maintain. Respondents noted that elderly clients need a homelike care environment, services based on age rather than on

TABLE 7-13

Perceived Differences between Elderly and Younger Mentally Retarded Persons in Institutionally Based Residential and Day Programs

TYPES OF DIFFERENCES	RESIDENTIAL (n = 140)	DAY (n = 62)	t
Physical health care	86.8%	78.9%	1.27
Different service needs	65.9	66.7	−.10
Preferences for activities	63.6	63.2	.05
Differences in energy levels	63.6	78.9	−2.23*
Differences in skill levels	48.1	26.6	2.96**
Motivation differences	38.8	40.4	−.20
Memory differences	38.8	40.4	−.20
Emotional/behavioral changes	27.9	38.6	−1.40
Friendship needs	22.5	35.1	−1.71
Desire for new skills	19.4	17.5	.30

$* = p<.05.$ $** = p<.01.$

their level of mental retardation, and more choice in their daily lives. Staff described the need to "scale down expectations" in designing programs, to include plenty of rest periods, and to anticipate that clients may become more withdrawn as they age. Interestingly, areas in the literature in which mentally retarded elders are assumed to exhibit differences associated with the aging process (i.e., motivation, memory, emotional needs) were less commonly noted by respondents as areas in which elderly mentally retarded persons were different from their younger counterparts.

Respondents were asked to describe the programmatic impacts associated with the unique or special needs of their elderly clients (see Table 7-14). The vast majority of both residential and day programs said that serving elderly clients affected their programmatic goals. The goals

TABLE 7-14

Programmatic Impacts of Special Needs of Institutionalized Elderly Mentally Retarded Persons

TYPES OF IMPACTS	RESIDENTIAL (n = 140)	DAY (n = 62)	t
Programmatic goals	76.0%	82.5%	−1.02
Duration of events	60.5	68.4	−1.05
Scheduling of events	57.4	66.7	−1.21
Design of age-appropriate activities	52.7	64.9	−1.57
Meeting health care needs	38.0	47.4	−1.18
Age range of programs	32.6	31.6	.13
Transportation needs	30.5	28.1	.33
Staffing	29.5	15.8	2.16*
Location of programs	27.9	33.3	−.73
Disability mix of participants	11.6	17.5	−1.02

$* = p<.05.$

most commonly affected by aging were socialization, maintenance of skills and health status, and provision of leisure time for hobbies. Many noted the need to be programmatically flexible and to encourage client choices. Virtually all said that program goals should be based on the individual's level of functioning.

Other commonly noted programmatic impacts were the duration and scheduling of events. Many respondents noted that events should span a shorter period than is typical and that fewer activities should be scheduled per session. Others noted that few evening activities were scheduled because clients were more likely to be too tired to participate.

Another major programmatic impact was the development of age-appropriate activities. Many noted that it is difficult to locate appropriate materials and that most staff had not worked with this age group previously. As their past training and experience were oriented towards younger mentally retarded persons, the degree of frustration for direct care staff and administrators in this regard was considerable.

Interestingly, fewer respondents noted impacts with respect to their staffing structures, age range, or disability mix of clients. However, some respondents noted that the location of the program assumes a critical importance. For example, it was important in some cases to have the program located on the first floor of the building and to have day programs located in close proximity to clients' residential programs. Transportation needs were also affected: vans with chairlifts were mentioned as a necessity by some respondents.

Finally, respondents were asked to project the types of changes that are likely to occur during the next two years with respect to either programmatic structure or client characteristics (see Table 7-15). The most frequently cited expected change noted by residential programs was in the disability level of their residents, which was expected to become more severe. Fewer residential programs foresaw an increase in the number of nonambulatory residents, in the number of more disabled residents, or a

TABLE 7-15

Programmatic Changes Anticipated by Institutionally Based Residential and Day Programs During Next Two Years

TYPE OF CHANGE	RESIDENTIAL ($n = 140$)	DAY ($n = 62$)	t
Disability level of clients	42.9%	41.9%	.12
Number of clients served	35.0	50.0	−1.98*
Physical facility design	27.1	41.9	−2.01*
Staffing	25.7	53.2	−3.72***
Age group served	22.1	16.1	1.02

* $= p<.05$.   *** $= p<.001$.

more mixed disability grouping of residents. Day programs projected changes in their staffing structure and ratio—most expressed the hope that more professional staff would be added to the program—as well as an increase in the number of elderly clients served and changes in the design of the physical facility.

RECOMMENDATIONS FOR
OTHER PROGRAMS

Respondents were asked what recommendations they might have for other programs regarding the structure, content, and orientation of programs for elderly mentally retarded person. Five major areas were covered in their recommendations. First, many respondents noted that a variety of community-based resources should/could be accessed. For example, one respondent advised that many communities have "garden clubs, civic and social clubs, hobby groups, etc." in which elderly mentally retarded persons could participate. Another recommended that service providers "visit other generic community programs and tie in with them instead of providing services in isolation."

A second area of recommendation pertained to the emphasis within programs on maintenance rather than acquisition of clients' skills. As respondents explained, for most institutionally based programs the dominant orientation is toward the enhancement or development of new skills in clients. A basic difference in institutionally based programs serving elderly mentally retarded persons is the need to substitute maintenance of skills or acquisition of new skills as a program goal.

A third topic on which recommendations were made was the importance of letting clients exercise preferences for different activities. One respondent noted, however, that providers have "to teach clients how to make choices." Another noted that in order to make choices clients need a range of activities from which to choose. This obviously requires that programs offer a variety of options and that the options change periodically.

A fourth set of recommendations related to staff training. Many respondents suggested that providers need training prior to initiation of the program. Most respondents coupled their recommendations about staff training to the issue of having accurate and complete knowledge about the clients' physical and medical status. The preparedness of staff to plan appropriate programs based on their understanding of the effects of aging was a commonly voiced concern for other programs. For example, one respondent said that staff have to "encourage the client to ask for help rather than always try to do things independently. Our clients have been encouraged over the past years to do everything as independently as they can. Now, as they are getting older, they have more physical difficulty in doing things but are sometimes hesitant to ask for help. That's where well trained staff are really important."

Finally, respondents had suggestions for the physical environment in which programs for the elderly are located. Many suggested that the size of the program be small and that the program space be physically accessible to persons with mobility impairments. One noted the importance of having a "quiet relaxation area rather than a large dayroom." Another offered that "temperature control is important."

These recommendations reflect the experiences of a diverse group of respondents in serving elderly mentally retarded persons in institutional settings. Interestingly, their recommendations were similar in scope and content to those reported by respondents of community-based programs (see Chapters 5 and 6). The thematic congruence of both institutionally based and community-based providers' recommendations regarding the manner in which programs for elderly mentally retarded persons should be structured and delivered suggests that it is possible to identify common principles of services for this group. These principles were: utilization of community resources, reorientation of programmatic emphasis on maintenance rather than acquisition of skills, exercise of clients choice, preparedness of staff, and physical modification of program space.

SUMMARY AND CONCLUSIONS

Institutionally based residential and day programs share both similarities and differences with each other. They tend to be similar in the types of clients served. In both residential and day programs, a majority of the clients are severely or profoundly retarded and are described as being in good or excellent health given their age and levels of disability. These clients also had similar patterns of additional disabilities. While the clients served in day programs were significantly older than those served in residential programs, the difference was only about 2 years (63.9 versus 61.8 years). The staff who were interviewed, whether they were from day or residential programs, expressed a common view of these clients and their needs. Few statistically significant differences between residential and day programs were found in respondents' views regarding the special issues they faced in serving elderly mentally retarded persons, the extent to which they perceived their elderly mentally retarded clients to be different from their younger mentally retarded clients, and the programmatic impacts of any special needs of the elderly client.

In contrast, differences were found between residential and day programs in structural characteristics. Day programs had begun more recently than had residential programs, and were more likely to have been developed specifically for the purpose of serving elderly mentally retarded clients. Day programs were larger, located in shared space, and sex-integrated, whereas residential programs were smaller, fully occupied their own buildings, and often served either men or women but not both. Finally, staff from residential and day programs differed in their expectations for programmatic changes during the next 2 years, with more changes expected by day program staff.

One paradoxical finding was that although about half of the clients were judged to be in good or excellent health for their ages and levels of disability, medical and health-related issues were paramount in the thoughts of the respondents. Specifically, many programs had entrance criteria based at least in part on clients' medical status. Nearly all day programs and more than one-third of the residential programs had nursing staff. When asked about staff training, the respondents reported that information about the physical aspects of aging was the most valuable content provided them. The most frequently reported special need of elderly as opposed to younger mentally retarded clients was their need for physical health care. Thus, although the institutionally based clients were not described as being in poor health as a group, the staff were very concerned about their health needs and medical status.

Chapter 8

Life Care
_____Communities
Programmatic
Prototypes

The purpose of this chapter is to describe six programs serving elderly mentally retarded persons that offered a comprehensive range of health, social, and residential services. These programs exhibited many similarities to the life care community model, an innovative comprehensive service model designed for the general elderly population. This chapter begins with a brief literature review about the life care community model and then examines the six programs that participated in the National Survey that bore similarities to this model.

BACKGROUND

It is commonly noted that the American system of health care (including service delivery mechanisms and the financing systems that support them) is more successful in providing acute care services than in providing long term care for chronically disabled or ill persons (Branch, 1987; Callahan & Wallack, 1981). While massive private and federal support underwrites medical services for the general population, persons with chronic disabilities (either from birth or from the consequences of accidents, illness, or aging) have neither the range of service delivery systems nor the financing structures to support their needs for residential, health, social, and support services. As Feinstein, Gornick, and Greenberg (1984) note, "the continuing disproportionate growth in health care expenditures, along with the problems surrounding the aging of the population and their long term care needs, are the major issues confronting the health care system today" (p. 7).

Given the absence of a national policy for addressing the long term care needs of chronically disabled persons, a variety of privately and publicly supported demonstration projects or models have evolved to test the feasibility of alternatives for persons with long term care needs (Feinstein, Gornick, Greenberg, 1984). These strategies include privately offered long term care insurance (Meiners, 1984), social/health mainte-

127

nance organization (Greenberg & Leutz, 1984), a variety of housing alternatives for the elderly (Gelwicks, 1984), home equity conversion to fund long term care services (Schloen, 1984), and programs to support family-based care (Cantor, 1984).

Among these rapidly growing developments in the long term care field is the "life care community", also known as a continuing care retirement community (Winklevoss & Powell, 1984). A life care community as described by Cohen (1980) is "a financially self-sufficient residential community for the elderly that offers medical and nursing services in specialized facilities on the premises. Its distinguishing feature—and the basis of its existence and operations—is a lifetime contract between the community and each resident that defines each party's financial and service obligations" (pp. 885–886). These communities have been historically linked to religious organizations that sought to establish a dignified setting in which elders could retain their independence while being assured of adequate and appropriate health care services in the event of declining capacities or illness. Residents pay an entrance fee to enter the community and monthly dues thereafter. In return, they are guaranteed that their social, health, and support needs will be met for the duration of their lives (Pies, 1984).

According to Ball (1983), there are approximately 275 life care communities in the country serving some 90,000 people. Further, these developments are relatively recent, with most having been established in the last decade by not-for-profit agencies (Bailey, 1983).

Life care communities represent a prototype for consideration by the field of mental retardation. However, their salient defining characteristics—up-front entrance fees and a comprehensive array of health, social, and support services—will require some reassessment and modification for use by mentally retarded persons. It is unlikely that any innovation in long term care for mentally retarded persons that requires a substantial up-front entrance fee will be effectively introduced, given the relative poverty of this group. However, the comprehensive array of services embodied in the life care communities presents a compelling model for meeting the needs of this population, particularly as they age and experience the inevitable declines associated with the aging process.

THE NATIONAL SURVEY

While many of the residential programs described earlier (see Chapters 5 and 7) possessed some of the characteristics of life care communities, the National Survey identified six specially designed programs that provided a continuum of health care services similar in structure and purpose to those offered in life care communities. The six programs to be described in this chapter were offered by four relatively large private residential facilities, with one facility operating three programs.

The programs were self-described as permanent retirement residential programs that enabled residents to live as independently as their functional abilities permitted with the back-up of skilled nursing care if needed. While they differed from traditional life care communities in their financing structures in that none required sizable up-front entrance fees, they were programmatically similar to life care communities. Each of the six programs is described below, followed by a summary of important attributes that may be useful in future deliberations about long term care options for elderly mentally retarded persons. All gave permission to be identified by name in this chapter.

CASE EXAMPLES

Marbridge Retirement Villa

The Marbridge Retirement Villa is a 52-bed facility that provides combined levels of nursing and retirement care for mentally retarded men and women. Its program was described as "specifically geared towards those mildly or moderately retarded persons who have reached the period of life that indicates retirement and/or nursing care." It is located in a rural, upper middle income neighborhood, 9 miles southwest of Austin, Texas, and it opened in October 1984. At the time of the Survey, the facility served 20 individuals (19 males and 1 female) ranging in age from 29 to 68. When they moved in, residents were encouraged to bring their private possessions with them because this was to become their permanent home. The double-occupancy bedrooms were large and each had its own bathroom. The common rooms included recreational areas for billiards and arts and crafts, a living room with a fireplace, a dining room, a pool, a sauna, exercise bikes, and an outdoor patio.

Exactly half (10) of the residents at Marbridge were 55 years of age or older. In order to be considered for admission, an individual had to be mentally retarded in the mild to moderate range, although severely retarded individuals who functioned in the moderate range were considered. Persons who were severely emotionally disturbed, who had other mental health problems, or who were stroke victims were not accepted. Applications from multiply handicapped persons were subjected to a special review. Each applicant's medical history was examined by a doctor and a nurse.

Of the 10 elderly mentally retarded individuals in the program at the time of the Survey, eight were moderately retarded and two were mildly retarded. There were nine males and one female. Further, eight were considered to be in good physical health while two were judged to be in fair health. Eight of these clients also had other disabilities such as epilepsy, visual impairments, hearing impairments, and diagnosed emotional problems.

Prior to their residence here, eight of the clients had lived at a training and care facility owned and operated by the agency sponsoring Marbridge Villa. One of the other two residents moved from a nursing home and the other came from an ICF/MR for 15 or fewer clients.

The goal of Marbridge Villa was to provide a comfortable atmosphere in which mentally retarded individuals could retire at an activity level of their own choosing. According to the administrator of the program, "activities" replaced work as the daytime activity. All of the elderly mentally retarded persons, then, spent the majority of their daytime hours at the residence, on residence-sponsored trips, or involved in various activities including arts and crafts, bowling, and taking trips to libraries, the beach, concerts, shows, etc. Residents were also paid for doing simple chores.

Other services that were provided included medical care (Level III care was available for those who needed it), nutritional advice, help with self care and basic skills, psychological counseling, and transportation in vehicles owned by the facility. None of the clients participated in any generic senior citizen programs in the outside community.

The staff supervising these activities included nine nurses (at least one of whom was on duty at all times), five dietary staff members, one administrator, and one direct care (nonnursing) staff member. One full-time person and one half-time person made up the maintenance staff and a physician and psychologist were available on a part-time basis. Seminars and workshops on nursing care, geriatrics, and the needs of the elderly mentally retarded were attended by staff members to train them to meet individualized client needs.

Overall, the administrator felt that the needs of the elderly mentally retarded clients were completely met by this program. His main concern, however, was about funding. As a private, nonprofit corporation, the facility's budget consisted of client tuition fees and gifts. As far as the future is concerned it was estimated that more staff would be needed within the year, as the total number of clients served was expected to increase from 20 to full capacity (52 individuals). It was also anticipated that these extra clients will have more acute medical needs than the present population.

St. Coletta School

St. Coletta was founded in 1904 by the Sisters of St. Francis of Assisi. Located in the rural farmlands of Jefferson, Wisconsin, the school has a residential capacity of 376 persons and also accepts day students. For each individual at the school, mental retardation must be the primary disability.

The aging mentally retarded clients lived in the school's Alverno Cottage, which was licensed as an intermediate care nursing home. Although the facility has served elderly mentally retarded adults since the late 1930s, a major expansion project began at Alverno in September, 1983. This resulted in the construction of modern semi-private residential rooms and bath facilities, a central dining room, and a modern chapel/auditorium. Programming in areas such as spiritual and social skills development, occupational therapy, physical activities, preventive health care, and recreational activities, was also increased. Finally, extra community involvement was encouraged through student and volunteer programs with area schools and universities. In order to offer this broad array of services, the Alverno project operated in 1984 on a budget of $700,000. Most of this money came from Medicaid, Medicare, SSDI, client fees, and special private grant funds.

The primary goal of the Alverno project was "to provide for continued spiritual growth and development of self-concept . . . through the provision of quality residential care and participation in meaningful daily programming activities." Each resident was allowed to choose the programs in which he or she wanted to participate and was encouraged to remain as active as possible. Through this program, the facility also hoped to "develop and promote a national model for the care of the aging developmentally disabled which allows for the best possible quality of life in a residential care setting."

At the time of the Survey, the Alverno Cottage housed 74 mentally retarded individuals ranging in age from 27 to 93. Thirty-nine were 55 years of age and above—12 of these were male and 27 female. The majority (28) were moderately retarded, while five were mildly and six were profoundly retarded. Some of the elderly mentally retarded clients also had secondary disabilities such as cerebral palsy or epilepsy, were nonambulatory or visually or hearing impaired, or had a diagnosed emotional problem. Overall, the facility administrator considered seven clients to be in excellent physical health while 17, 11, and four were judged to be in good, fair, and poor health, respectively.

Prior to living at Alverno, most of the residents had been in a different program at St. Coletta. Three had lived at home with their families and one had moved from a nursing home. As retirees, 36 of the elderly mentally retarded residents spent most of their time at the cottage involved in formal programming. In contrast, three clients worked in a transitional employment setting. None of the clients, however, participated in any of the generic senior citizen programs provided in the community. Overall, the facility administrator felt that the needs of the elderly mentally retarded were completely met by the St. Coletta program.

The professional staff at Alverno consisted of one administrator, 18 direct care (nonnursing) staff, two occupational therapists, one full-time and one half-time nurse, and one half-time social worker. A variety of consultants (such as a psychologist, speech therapist, pharmacist, and dietician) were available. Further, medical and dental professionals were accessible by the program. In order to prepare them better to serve the needs of the elderly mentally retarded persons, staff members were provided with written materials, attended outside seminars and workshops, and received in-service training.

As for the future, the School is dedicated to making the 1980s "a decade devoted to adult education and programming." Toward this end there will be an increased use of volunteers, more transportation to encourage integration with the community, and additional improvements to the physical plant. Clients will continue to be asked about their wishes and preferences and the religious development of residents will also continue to be emphasized.

The Woods School

The Woods School and Residential Treatment Center provides comprehensive educational, social, and clinical services in residential and day programs for children and adults with mental retardation, brain damage, neurological impairment, learning disabilities, multiple handicaps, deafness, and cerebral palsy. Established in 1921, the campus covers 300 acres and is located 20 miles north of Philadelphia in the town of Langhorne. More than 580 residents and approximately 20 day students were enrolled in the Woods School at the time of the Survey.

In August 1981, a decision was made to develop a program to serve older mentally retarded clients. No special funding was received to start this program. It was developed out of the school's overall budget, which lists as its sources, Medicaid, SSI, Social Security, and private funding. The retirement residence for men and women became known as Birchwood. The one-story building had two bedroom wings, one each for the men and the women. It also had dining, living, recreation, and activity rooms as well as a family-style kitchen that encouraged independent eating choices. Fifteen mentally retarded individuals between the ages of 59 and 74 lived in this unit. Their level of functioning varied—five were mildly retarded, seven were moderately retarded, and three were profoundly retarded. In addition, many of them had a secondary disability such as cerebral palsy, visual or hearing impairment, or a diagnosed emotional problem. Overall, however, the director of the program considered four of them to be in excellent physical health and six in good health, while four were judged to be in fair health and one in poor physical health. Prior to moving to Birchwood, all of these individuals had lived at home with their families.

One goal of this program was to create a balance between self-directed leisure time and staff-supervised activities. Many of the clients participated in generic senior citizen programs offered in the community. The staff and other seniors involved in these programs were generally very receptive to the elderly mentally retarded participants. Overall, the director felt that the needs of this population were nearly completely met at Birchwood.

The Birchwood staff had been specially trained in working with elderly mentally retarded persons through seminars, workshops, and classes in CPR and first aid. The staff consisted of one full-time and one part-time administrator, seven full-time and one half-time direct care (nonnursing) workers, one half-time nurse, and a part-time psychologist and social worker.

The director's special concerns focused on the need for additional residences and day programs to more fully serve elderly mentally retarded persons. He also felt that retirement programs needed appropriate back-up medical services. In addition, he noted that one should "never assume because people are getting older that they can't become more independent. There is still room for growth and development."

Elwyn Institutes

Elwyn Institutes is a comprehensive rehabilitation facility serving 630 individuals on a campus that consists of 22 separate buildings. The clients served include those with mental retardation as well as those with mental health problems, head trauma, blindness, deafness, and physical disabilities. Located 14 miles southwest of Philadelphia, Elwyn Institutes has been in operation since 1852. New buildings have been added over the years to increase space and the older units have been converted to other uses. A vast array of services is provided including individualized active treatment programming, nursing and nutritional services, physical, occupational, and speech therapy, recreational and social activities, psychological counseling, social work services, and transportation services.

At the time of the National Survey, there were three residential sites serving the elderly population. The clients in each residence spent most of their weekday hours in one of the three specialized day programs for elderly clients. The particular day program was determined by the clients' needs, the clients' interests, and recommendations of the Interdisciplinary Team. In addition, continued programming occurred in the clients' residential living area as supported by residential, recreational, and ancillary staff. Although little use was made of the generic senior citizen programs offered in nearby communities, there was an emphasis on utilizing community resources.

Overall, Elwyn Institutes believed programming was enhanced through seminars and workshops for staff. Specific training was provided in the areas of the aging process, legal issues, abuse, death and dying, and individualization of programming. In the section that follows, the characteristics of each of the three residences are described, followed by a general overview of special concerns and thoughts about the future.

North Hall occupied the second floor of the one self-contained building with its own dining room and living/recreational areas. Although it had a capacity to serve 48 individuals, only 41 clients lived there at the time of the National Survey. All were mentally retarded and ranged in age from 35 to 103. The majority were moderately to severely retarded, while seven functioned in the mild range and seven others functioned in the profoundly retarded range. Thirty clients—19 males and 11 females—were age 55 and older. Many of the elderly mentally retarded clients also had other disabilities, including cerebral palsy, epilepsy, mobility problems, visual and/or hearing losses, and language problems. Two elderly clients were judged to be in excellent physical health, while 19 were considered to be in good or fair health and nine were judged to be in poor health. The staff for this residence consisted of one administrator, four supervisors, 27 direct care (nonnursing) staff, and two nurses. Additional support staff included physicians, therapists, a social worker, a psychologist, a recreational therapist, and instructional staff.

Smith Hall was a residential hall with a total capacity of 79 individuals. At the time of the Survey, there were 65 residents—28 males and 37 females. The majority were considered moderately retarded, while 15 were considered mildly retarded and 10 profoundly retarded. All residents except for one male and two females were age 55 and above. Several residents had other disabilities as well, including cerebral palsy, epilepsy, ambulation difficulties, and visual and/or hearing losses. Twenty-six residents were considered to be in excellent or good physical health, while 36 were judged to be in fair physical health. Staff included two administrators, four supervisors, 33 direct care (nonnursing) staff, two nurses, two social workers, and one psychologist, as well as the support staff previously indicated.

Maris Hall, at the time of the Survey was a 60-bed residence for 51 clients ranging in age from 33 to 90. There were 33 elderly mentally retarded individuals—13 males and 20 females. The majority were considered mildly retarded and only a few had secondary disabilities. Fourteen individuals were judged to be in good physical health, 16 were in fair health, and only three were in poor health. Maris Hall was staffed with one administrator, four supervisors, 24 direct care (nonnursing) staff, one social worker, a psychologist, and the other support staff as identified earlier.

In the future, Elwyn Institutes expected that these three residential programs will continue to adapt to client needs. The programmatic orientation was described as including clients in ongoing activities, focusing on increasing—or at the very least maintaining—the clients' skills and abilities, and increasing the amount of relevant in-service training provided to staff.

CONCLUSIONS

Although none of the six facilities referred to its program as a life care community, each created a long term care option in order to respond to the needs of elderly mentally retarded persons. While there were some clear similarities across the six programs—notably, the provision of the full range of needed services rather than one component only—there were also some important distinctions.

For example, five facilities had developed the aging program to meet the needs of their own residents who had reached old age (Marbridge, St. Coletta, and the three Elwyn Institutes residences), while one primarily served elderly residents who had previously lived elsewhere (Woods School). The residents of one facility (Woods School) actively participated in community-based generic senior citizen programs, while the others were largely self-contained.

Interestingly, one program (Elwyn Institutes) encouraged the residents to develop new skills. This is a comparatively unusual goal for programs serving elderly mentally retarded persons, where the maintenance of skills and development of leisure time activities tend to be emphasized instead. Only one facility (Woods School) exclusively served elderly mentally retarded persons, while the others served a chronologically mixed age group, although the programs were self-designated as serving the elderly. Finally, one served primarily moderately or mildly retarded persons (Marbridge), while the other three served a more varied range of cognitively impaired residents.

These differences and commonalties across the six facilities raise several questions regarding the provision of services to elderly mentally retarded persons in facilities similar to life care communities. For one, these programs were clearly out of the mainstream of urban community living. Each was located in a rural area and was set on a campus. They also tended to be somewhat larger than either the community-based or the institutionally-based residential programs described in Chapters 5 and 7. It is important to keep in mind, however, that many nonretarded elders also live in retirement communities that are often set in rural areas on large, self-contained campuses. Despite their similarity with retirement communities, it may be legitimate to call these programs private institutions. To what extent do life care communities and private institutions share common characteristics? To what extent do they share common effects?

Further, each of the six facilities provided a comprehensive array of services to clients, including medical, social, and habilitative as well as residential support. Like life care communities, all such resources were present within the facility. What are the costs and benefits of creating such a self-contained community?

Third, placement in one of these facilities represents a distinct alternative for elderly mentally retarded persons to more mainstream programs. The six programs were intended to provide a permanent home for residents and were thus responsive to families' concerns about security and future stability. While these facilities' aging units had only been operating for a short while at the time of the National Survey, it is possible that some residents will live in these life care communities for 20 or 30 years. During these years, the residents' service needs will fluctuate and intensify, especially within the medical domain. Future research should track the differential potential of this type of program as compared with community-based and public institutional programs to effectively respond to the needs of aging mentally retarded persons and to create a desirable quality of life for them.

Issues in the Provision of Services to Elderly Mentally Retarded Persons

Chapter 9

Utilization of
_____Senior Centers

BACKGROUND

During the upcoming years it will be increasingly common for elderly mentally retarded persons to be served by programs and services within the aging network. This pattern of generic service utilization is consistent with the larger trend toward increased integration of mentally retarded persons into society at large. Since the early 1970s, it has become more and more common for mentally retarded persons to be served in integrated settings rather than in segregated settings (Lakin & Bruininks, 1985). Just as mentally retarded children are now mainstreamed in public schools and mentally retarded adults often live in community-based residential settings, some mentally retarded elders are now served by the generic aging network. Mentally retarded persons aged 60 or older are eligible for the generic services authorized by the Older Americans Acts by virtue of age alone.

Another factor that will motivate utilization of the generic aging network by elderly mentally retarded persons pertains to the limited availability of informal supports for this group. Gerontological research has clearly demonstrated an inverse relationship between the availability of informal supports and the need for formal support services (Brody, 1985). Persons with limited informal supports tend to be heavy service users. Because aging mentally retarded persons generally do not have children or spouses on whom they can depend for support, their family network at best consists of very old parents, aging siblings, and the children of siblings. As we noted in Chapter 2, little is known about the quality of sibling relationships over the full life cycle in families with a mentally retarded member. The willingness of siblings to provide informal support to their mentally retarded brothers and sisters in adulthood and old age remains to be examined. For all of these reasons, elderly mentally retarded persons may have a sharply reduced level of informal support available to them as compared with their age peers in the general population (Seltzer, 1985). A likely consequence is that mentally retarded elders will utilize formal services at a much higher rate than does the general elderly population.

As we noted in Chapter 1, there are three routes by which elderly mentally retarded persons obtain formal services. These are: participation in programs for younger mentally retarded adults (the *age-integration option*); participation in specialized programs for elderly mentally retarded persons such as those described in Chapters 5, 6, 7, and 8 (the *specialized service option*); and participation in programs for nonhandicapped elderly persons (the *generic services integration option*).

In this chapter, we will examine the extent to which elderly mentally retarded persons who participate in specialized services offered primarily through the mental retardation service system also utilize the generic services integration option.

THE GENERIC SERVICES
INTEGRATION OPTION

In the generic services integration option, elderly mentally retarded persons are included in services designed for the general (that is, nonretarded) elderly population. This is probably the least frequently utilized service option, although undoubtedly there are many mentally retarded elders not currently known to the mental retardation service system who participate "invisibly" in generic aging services.

In one of the only studies to examine this service option, Seltzer and Wells (1986) interviewed the directors of generic senior centers in Boston that currently provide services to mentally retarded elders. They found that staff in these programs were highly supportive of the policy of serving mentally retarded elders along with their nonretarded elderly clients and that there was a record of successful integration of the two client groups.

Although these findings are encouraging, the feasibility and appropriateness of integrating elderly mentally retarded persons into generic senior centers is largely a function of the extent to which the elderly mentally retarded and the elderly nonretarded participants share common characteristics and needs. High functioning elderly mentally retarded persons may be excellent candidates for mainstreaming into generic senior centers. Such individuals generally compare favorably with nonretarded elderly persons, who may have serious chronic illnesses or cognitive and functional limitations. Thus, the diagnosis of mental retardation alone should not be seen as a barrier to utilization of generic aging services. Rather, the mentally retarded person's functional abilities, interests, and service needs and the service capacities of the generic aging program should determine whether utilization of the generic services integration option is desirable in each case.

There are several ways in which elderly mentally retarded persons can be integrated into generic senior centers. First, individual elderly mentally retarded persons may participate in such programs with no special assistance, structure, or identification. No estimate of the prevalence of such participation or its success is available. Second, a group of elderly mentally retarded persons may participate *as a group* in a generic senior center. A number of such programs were identified in the National Survey and were described in Chapters 5 (mixed residential programs) and 6 (senior citizens programs). It is often the case in such programs that the elderly mentally retarded persons are seen as a distinct subgroup within the larger program, with special supports provided to them by the program. As we noted in Chapter 6, it was very common for the agencies that sponsored senior citizens programs also to operate programs that primarily served mentally retarded persons. Thus, there was an unusually high level of structural integration of the formal aging and mental retardation service systems represented in such agencies, which undoubtedly facilitated the participation of mentally retarded elders in generic aging programs.

The third way in which elderly mentally retarded persons can utilize generic senior centers is for staff from specialized programs for elderly mentally retarded persons to arrange for their participation and, often, to accompany their clients to the generic senior center. While in the second option it was the senior center program that provided the special supports to elderly mentally retarded participants, in this option such supports are provided by the mental retardation service system. In the National Survey, we examined the extent to which staff from specialized programs serving elderly mentally retarded persons had utilized generic senior centers on behalf of their clients. Our findings are presented below.

UTILIZATION OF GENERIC
SENIOR CENTERS BY
COMMUNITY-BASED
PROGRAMS

Figure 9-1 depicts the use of generic senior centers by community-based residential and day programs for elderly mentally retarded persons. Omitted from these analyses were the six specialized programs discussed in Chapter 8 and the 16 senior citizens programs that participated in the National Survey (see Chapter 6). Thus, the 305 programs included in these analyses can be characterized as specialized community-based programs for elderly mentally retarded persons that utilized generic senior centers to one degree or another.

We found that among community-based programs, it is the norm rather than the exception for specialized programs serving elderly mentally retarded persons to have accessed generic senior centers on behalf of their clients. As shown in Figure 9-1, nearly 60% of the

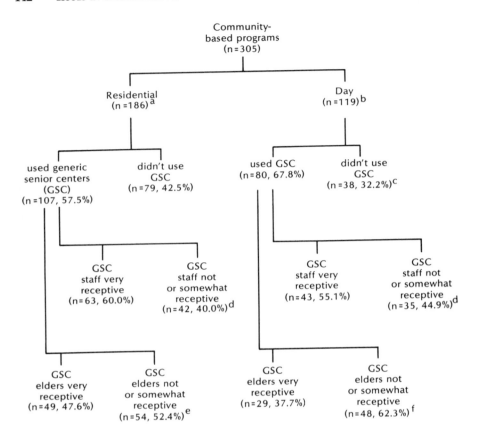

a The six programs discussed in Chapter 8 were omitted from these analyses.
b Programs included in the senior citizens program model from the Day Program typology
   were omitted from these analyses (n = 16).
c Missing data for 1 program.
d Missing data for 2 programs.
e Missing data for 4 programs.
f Missing data for 3 programs.

FIGURE 9-1:   Use of Generic Senior Centers by Community Programs (N = 305)

community-based residential and nearly 70% of the community-based day programs had utilized generic senior centers at least once on behalf of their elderly mentally retarded clients.

The level of generic service utilization depicted in Figure 9-1 suggests that a large number of staff from specialized services for elderly mentally retarded persons have interacted with the generic aging network on behalf of their clients. These staff, who often accompanied clients to the generic programs, have been repeatedly exposed to services included within the aging network. Thus, there has been a considerable amount of interaction among the two service sectors at the grassroots level.

CHARACTERISTICS OF
PROGRAMS THAT UTILIZED
GENERIC SENIOR CENTERS

What types of community-based residential and day programs utilized generic senior centers on behalf of their clients? Significant differences between programs that did and those that did not have at least one client participating in generic senior centers are presented in Table 9-1.

Community-Based Residential Programs

As shown in Table 9-1, community-based residential programs that utilized generic senior centers were significantly more likely to be sponsored by private nonprofit agencies than were programs that did not utilize such centers on behalf of their clients. They were also more likely to provide training to their staff on aging and mental retardation, which perhaps facilitated the staff's interaction with the generic senior centers. In addition to training, the composition of the staff in specialized programs for elderly mentally retarded persons may have made utilization of generic aging networks on behalf of their clients more feasible. These programs were significantly more likely to have had at least one administrator, one direct care staff member, and one teacher than were programs that did not utilize generic senior centers, but were less likely to have at least one homemaker. Administrators, direct care staff, and teachers may accompany elderly mentally retarded clients to generic senior centers, whereas homemakers are unlikely to do so.

The services provided by community-based residential programs that utilized generic senior centers on behalf of their clients differed in several respects from the services provided by programs that did not. The former type of program offered a significantly greater number of social/day services to their residents, were more likely to provide legal assistance services to them, and had a smaller percentage of their residents remain at home during the day with no formal in-home program.

In sum, utilization of generic senior centers was more common in community-based residential programs that were sponsored by nonprofit agencies, that had staff who could accompany clients to generic senior

TABLE 9-1

Utilization of Generic Senior Centers by Community-Based Residential
and Day Programs (N = 304)

| | UTILIZATION OF GENERIC SENIOR CENTERS | | |
	YES	NO	
A. *Community-Based Residential Programs*	(n = 107)	(n = 79)	t
1. Sponsorship of program (percent nonprofit)	56	41	2.11*
2. Percent providing special staff training about aging and MR	74	51	3.19**
3. Percent programs with at least 1 administrator	96	87	2.13*
4. Percent programs with at least 1 direct care staff member	95	86	2.09*
5. Percent programs with at least 1 homemaker	6	20	−2.89**
6. Percent programs with at least 1 teacher	14	4	2.55*
7. Number of social/day services provided to EMR residents	1.25	1.09	1.92*
8. Percent programs providing legal assistance to EMR clients	24	11	2.34*
9. Percent EMR who spend the day at the residence with no formal day program	13	25	−2.25*
B. *Community-Based Day Programs*	(n = 80)	(n = 38)	t
1. First year day program served EMR clients	1982	1980	2.34*
2. Percent day programs created to serve EMR clients	66	37	3.11**
3. Percent received special funds during first year of operation	34	16	1.98*
4. Percent received special funds during any year of operation	42	24	1.97*
5. Percent programs providing transportation services to EMR clients	88	66	2.51*
6. Percent of clients in day program aged 61–69	40	29	2.95**
7. Percent of clients in day program who live with their family	10	5	2.45*
8. Percent of clients in day program who live in semi-independent apartments	4	1	2.45*

* = $p < .05$.   ** = $p < .01$.

centers, and that provided more social and recreational services to their clients.

Community-Based Day Programs

Community-based day programs that utilized generic senior centers on behalf of their clients had begun operation more recently than had day programs that did not utilize generic senior centers (1982 vs. 1980). Day programs that utilized generic senior centers were more likely to have been created specifically to provide services to elderly mentally retarded persons, to receive special funding to support their services, and to provide transportation services than were programs that did not access generic aging services for their clients. These differences suggest that recently developed community-based day programs that were begun for the expressed purpose of serving the elderly mentally retarded population and that had transportation services were more likely to interact with the generic aging network than were those programs that did not receive special funding, that evolved into serving elderly mentally retarded persons as their clients aged, or that did not have the capacity for transporting clients.

There were also differences in the client populations served by day programs that did and did not access generic senior centers. A higher proportion of clients in community-based day programs that utilized generic senior centers were between the ages of 61 and 69 than clients in programs that did not. Also, a higher percentage of clients in the day programs that utilized generic aging programs lived with their families and in semi-independent apartments than clients in programs that did not. Thus, living in a more integrated or normalized residential setting was associated with utilization of generic seniors centers.

UTILIZATION OF GENERIC SENIOR CENTERS BY INSTITUTIONALLY BASED PROGRAMS

Figure 9-2 depicts the use of generic senior centers by institutionally based residential and day programs for elderly mentally retarded persons. In comparison with community-based programs, the utilization rate of institutionally based programs was much lower—approximately 25%. Yet, it was encouraging to find even this number of both residential and day programs in public institutions that had taken at least one client to a generic senior center in the community.

Institutionally Based Residential Programs

A number of interesting characteristics differentiate institutionally based programs that utilized generic senior centers from those that did not (see Table 9-2). Residential programs that accessed generic senior centers on behalf of their clients were significantly more likely to have at least one teacher and at least one recreational staff member than were programs that did not take their clients to senior centers. Importantly, residential settings that utilized generic senior centers provided their clients with a fuller pro-

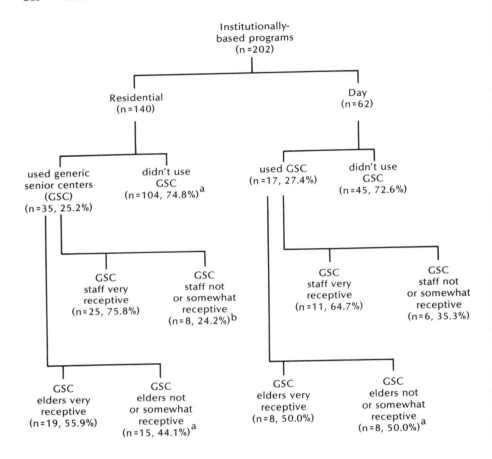

a Missing data for 1 program.
b Missing data for 2 programs.

FIGURE 9-2:   Use of Generic Senior Centers by Institutionally Based Programs
(N = 202)

gram of activities than those that did not, as measured by the frequency
with which 25 activities (such as social skills training, nutritional education
programs, and gardening) were scheduled. Thus, programmatic richness
was associated with utilization of generic senior centers.

The residents of institutionally based programs that utilized generic
senior centers were, on the average, older, more cognitively able, and less
likely to be in poor health than were those who lived in institutionally

TABLE 9-2

Utilization of Generic Senior Centers by Institutionally Based Programs (N = 202)

	UTILIZATION OF GENERIC SENIOR CENTERS		
	YES	NO	
A. *Institutionally Based Residential Programs*	(n = 35)	(n = 104)	t
1. Percent programs with at least 1 teacher	49	22	3.07**
2. Percent programs with at least 1 recreation staff member	91	75	2.56*
3. Total number activities provided to EMR residents (of list of 25 activities)	14.26	12.38	2.07*
4. Number activities provided to EMR residents occasionally (out of 25)	2.34	1.64	2.11*
5. Number activities never provided to EMR residents (out of 25)	9.94	12.16	−2.43*
6. Percent of residents aged 22–50	11	17	−1.99*
7. Percent of EMR residents who are mildly retarded	24	12	2.56*
8. Percent of EMR residents who are severely or profoundly retarded	54	72	−3.28***
9. Percent of EMR residents in poor health	7	12	−2.41*
10. Percent of EMR residents who spend the day at the residence in a formal day program	12	24	−2.07*
B. *Institutionally Based Day Programs*	(n = 17)	(n = 45)	t
1. Number clients in day program aged 55 or older	41.06	26.00	2.06*
2. Percent programs with at least one recreation staff member	82	47	2.63*
3. Number activities provided occasionally to EMR clients (out of a list of 25 activities)	16.00	13.27	2.39*
4. Number activities provided to EMR clients on a weekly basis (out of 25)	7.24	4.64	2.72**
5. Number activities never provided to EMR clients (out of 25)	8.53	11.13	−2.29*
6. Percent of EMR clients who are mildly retarded	19	7	2.89**
7. Percent of EMR clients who are moderately retarded	29	12	2.64*
8. Percent of EMR clients who are severely or profoundly retarded	52	81	−3.93***

* = $p<.05$.   ** = $p<.01$.   *** = $p<.001$.

based programs that did not utilize generic senior centers. Further, a smaller percentage of residents in programs that utilized generic senior centers spent their days at the residential unit in formal day programs.

Institutionally Based Day Programs

Differences between institutionally based day programs that utilized generic senior centers and those that did not are parallel to differences between residential programs of these two types (see Table 9-2). Specifically, day programs that took their clients to senior centers were significantly more likely to have at least one recreation specialist on staff, to have scheduled a greater number of activities for clients, and to serve more intellectually capable clients than were day programs that did not access generic senior centers. Further, programs that utilized generic senior centers had a significantly greater number of clients enrolled who were aged 55 or older.

In sum, in both residential and day institutionally based programs, utilization of generic senior centers was more likely when certain conditions and resources were in place, including: having a recreation specialist on staff; having a varied and full schedule of activities for clients; and having clients who were more intellectually capable and therefore presumably able to interact more successfully with the elders they encounter at the senior centers.

RECEPTIVITY OF GENERIC SENIOR CENTERS

How receptive are staff from the generic senior centers to the participation of mentally retarded elders? How receptive are the nonretarded elders? As shown in Figures 9-1 and 9-2, the majority of respondents in both institutionally based and community-based day and residential programs rated staff from generic senior centers as "very receptive" to the participation of mentally retarded elders and between one-third and one-half of the respondents rated the nonhandicapped elders as "very receptive". Thus, the integration process, at least as reported by staff of specialized programs for elderly mentally retarded persons, has had a favorable beginning.

What are the factors associated with staff and elderly clients from senior centers welcoming the participation of elderly mentally retarded clients? We conducted a series of analyses in order to determine whether programs that reported encountering "very receptive" staff and elders at senior centers differed from programs that reported encountering "somewhat" or "not at all" receptive staff and elders.

No consistent pattern of differences between these two types of programs were found with respect to the structural characteristics of the programs, the activities they provided, or their staff. However, some characteristics of the elderly mentally retarded clients were associated with a more receptive welcome from senior center staff and clients. These are summarized in Tables 9-3 and 9-4. These data suggest that staff from generic seniors centers are more receptive to the participation of elderly mentally retarded persons who are older and in better health. Elders from senior centers seem to be more receptive to the participation of younger and healthier elderly mentally retarded persons.

TABLE 9-3

Client Characteristics Associated with Reported Receptivity of Staff from Generic Seniors Centers

	STAFF VERY RECEPTIVE		
	YES	NO	
I. *Community-Based Programs*			
A. *Residential Programs*	$(n = 63)$	$(n = 42)$	t
1. Average level of health of EMR clients[a]	1.97	1.76	2.09*
B. *Day Programs*	$(n = 43)$	$(n = 35)$	t
1. Percent of clients aged 61–69	35	45	−2.26*
II. *Institutionally Based Programs*			
A. *Residential Programs*	$(n = 25)$	$(n = 8)$	t
1. Percent of clients aged 55 or older	83	69	2.01*
2. Percent of clients aged 22–50	9	19	−2.26*
3. Percent of clients aged 70 or older	30	17	2.11*
B. *Day Programs* — no differences			

[a] Coded as 3 = excellent, 2 = good, 1 = fair, 0 = poor, per judgments of the respondents.
* = $p < .05$.

TABLE 9-4

Client Characteristics Associated with Reported Receptivity by Elders from Generic Seniors Centers

	ELDERS VERY RECEPTIVE		
	YES	NO	
I. *Community-Based Programs*			
A. *Residential Programs*	$(n = 49)$	$(n = 54)$	t
Percent of clients aged 55–60	28	20	1.97*
B. *Day Programs*	$(n = 29)$	$(n = 48)$	t
1. Percent of EMR clients in good health[a]	62	43	2.69**
2. Percent of EMR clients in poor health[a]	6	12	−2.15*
II. *Institutionally Based Programs*			
A. *Residential Programs*	$(n = 19)$	$(n = 15)$	t
Percent of clients who are moderately retarded	15	32	3.55***
B. *Day Programs*	$(n = 8)$	$(n = 8)$	t
Average age of clients	61.30	67.61	−2.49*

[a] Coded as 3 = excellent, 2 = good, 1 = fair, 0 = poor, per judgments of the respondents.
* = $p < .05$. ** = $p < .01$. *** = $p < .001$.

CONCLUSIONS

Although there was a considerable amount of participation in generic senior centers by elderly mentally retarded persons from specialized residential and day programs in both community-based and institutionally based settings, it would be inappropriate to conclude that such participation is necessarily desirable or feasible for all elderly mentally retarded persons or for all programs that serve them. It has become a truism in the field of mental retardation that no one service is equally appropriate for all mentally retarded persons given the heterogeneity of the population of service recipients. This is also true with respect to the utilization of the generic aging network by elderly mentally retarded persons. The findings presented in this chapter provide some guidelines as to when utilization is most feasible and when it will be met with support from the staff and elders from the senior centers.

It seems that the characteristics of the *program* are predictive of whether staff will utilize a generic senior center on behalf of clients, while the characteristics of the *clients* are predictive of whether their participation will be welcomed by staff and elders from the senior center. Salient program characteristics predictive of utilization can be classified as those that either defined the program as an aging service (created rather than evolved, having received special funding, offering special staff training on aging) or that created the capacity for the program to interact with the aging network (staff, transportation). Salient client characteristics predictive of the extent to which staff and elders from senior centers welcomed the participation of elderly mentally retarded persons included the age and reported health status of the elders with mental retardation. Both staff and elders were seen as more receptive when the elderly mentally retarded persons were healthier. However, whereas staff were more receptive when the mentally retarded clients were older, elders were more receptive when the mentally retarded persons were younger.

The overall conclusions we have drawn from these findings are that participation in the generic aging network is possible for elderly mentally retarded persons, that it is a fairly widespread phenomenon, and that a favorable experience is commonly reported. More research is needed in order to explore fully the implications of these patterns and to examine the long range effects of the generic services integration option on the elderly mentally retarded persons and on the staff and elders from the generic senior centers.

Chapter 10

Retirement
Options

BACKGROUND

Among the issues frequently raised regarding elderly mentally retarded persons are the positive and negative consequences of their retirement from structured, typically vocationally oriented day programs. A wide range of perspectives are expressed by professionals on this issue. Some are of the opinion that mentally retarded persons should not retire (Wolfensberger, 1985). The inference is that retirement is equated with the cessation of purposeful, guided activity. These professionals fear that if mentally retarded people retire, they will become passive, their skills will regress, and they will face idle, unstimulating days. Continued participation in active treatment programs is, according to this view, considered to be as desirable in old age as in earlier stages of life.

Other professionals are of the opinion that retirement options should exist for mentally retarded persons as they do for other older persons (Catapano, Levy, & Levy, 1985). The inference is that as mentally retarded persons age, their interest in and endurance capacities for participating in vocationally and/or educationally oriented day programs wanes. It is expected that alternative programs, either full- or part-time, should be available that allow persons to engage in varied leisure activities that do not require the same stamina nor have the traditional expectations of skill development and active treatment that are characteristic of regular day programs.

Implicit in each of these perspectives is the realization that the issue of retirement for mentally retarded persons has consequences for policy development, for service provision, and for the elderly individual with mental retardation. The purpose of this chapter is to explore the policy and programmatic implications of retirement for this population.

The chapter begins with a brief discussion of retirement for the general population. Issues such as the role of retirement in the life span of the individual, the trend toward early retirement, the social and economic rationales for retirement, and the factors influencing individual decision making regarding retirement are reviewed. The chapter then presents data from the National Survey regarding the extent to which retirement options exist and are exercised by elderly mentally retarded persons in a variety of age-specialized community-based residential programs. The general and specific problems faced by programs regarding retirement issues are discussed.

It should be noted that the data reported in this chapter were collected from programs in which a substantial number (at least 50%) of mentally retarded participants were age 55 or older. Thus, these programs were directly facing the positive and negative consequences of retirement decisions for their clients. The insights, attitudes, and opinions of the respondents grew out of the direct experiences of staff faced with the challenge of meeting the day program needs of elderly mentally retarded clients.

RETIREMENT FOR THE NONRETARDED AGING POPULATION

Studies indicate that there has been a substantial increase in the number of years during an individual's lifetime that are devoted to retirement. For example, the US Senate Special Committee on Aging reported that "compared to a century ago, children are spending more time in school, both men and women in their middle years are spending more time in work, and older people are spending more time in retirement" (1985–1986 edition, p. 71). In 1900, the average length of retirement was 1.2 years. In 1980, an average of 13.8 years were spent in retirement. Thus, retirement has become a major phase in the individual life cycle (Neugarten & Hagestad, 1976).

Contrary to stereotypic views of retirement, it is not an event that the majority of those in the labor force wish to postpone as long as possible. Ironically, as the mandatory retirement age crept up from 65 to 70 (and was subsequently repealed altogether for most federal employees in 1978), the percentage of the American labor force who were retiring early (before mandatory retirement age) steadily increased. As Robinson, Coberly, and Paul (1985) noted, "The decline in labor force participation rates of males over the age of 55 in the last several decades is the major phenomenon to be noted in the employment status of older persons" (p. 504). Their analysis indicates that in 1981, 11% of the civilian labor force were men and women between the ages of 55 and 64. By 1995, it is expected that this cohort will comprise only 8.6% of the civilian labor force. This is attributed both to the declining labor force participation of older persons and to the growth in the prime age segments of the work force.

It has been argued that the social and economic purposes of retirement have shifted as well. Atchley (1982) noted that the concept of retirement is no longer firmly linked to the concept of old age. Retirement used to be rationalized as a means of gracefully shedding workers deemed no longer fit to work because of their age-related declines in productivity. It now serves as a mechanism "to control unemployment and creation of job opportunities . . . the issue (is) less the effect of aging and more the need to circulate a large labor force through a somewhat smaller array of jobs" (Atchley, 1982, p. 274).

While retirement is commonly viewed as an abrupt, total departure from the labor force, it can also be a *process* by which an individual gradually or partially withdraws from an employment situation (Atchley, 1982; Robinson, Coberly, & Paul, 1985). Indeed, the likelihood of working on a part-time basis increases with age. The results of national surveys (Louis Harris and Associates, Inc., 1979) showed clear preferences for part-time work among older persons. This was especially true for persons employed full-time who were interested in post-retirement employment. Other reasons why part-time work is more common among older citizens are disability, illness, or layoffs (Axel & Brotman, 1982; Rones, 1978).

The decision to retire represents one of the most important choices an individual makes. Whether viewed as a conscious tradeoff between work and leisure (as conceptualized by labor economists) or as an exchange of social roles (as conceptualized by sociologists), the decision to retire marks a major transition point for the individual within his or her life development.

A variety of empirical studies have investigated the factors that influence the decision to retire. As Robinson, Coberly, and Paul (1985) noted, these studies have identified both individual and institutional factors related to the decisionmaking process. Studies of persons who retired early (before age 65) found that poorer health and having an adequate retirement income were the two major factors contributing to early retirement (Barfield & Morgan, 1969; Schulz, 1980). Further, persons who preferred less work and who had a positive image of retirement were more likely to retire early (Barfield & Morgan, 1969; Orbach, 1969). Institutionally based factors relating to retirement decisions include the availability of flexible work schedules for older persons (McConnell, Fleisher, Usher, & Kaplan, 1980), pension plan policies (Schulz, 1983), and general labor market conditions (Clark & Barker, 1981).

These trends and issues have important implications for the study of retirement options for elderly mentally retarded persons. First, retirement does not necessarily mean the abrupt cessation of one's current employment situation. Retirement may well be a process, spanning several years, in which a gradual shift in the individual's work schedule and activities occurs. Second, retirement does not necessarily mean the termination of employment. Many persons in the general population move from full-time to part-time employment after they have officially retired. Third, the percentage of older citizens in the labor force is declining. Thus, retirement is becoming a predictable and often positively anticipated life stage that offers the opportunity for an expansion of leisure and recreation time. Finally, the ability of employers to encourage or tolerate early retirement among the work force provides wider opportunities for the remaining work force. This may act as a safety valve for the job aspirations of the baby boom generation among mentally retarded persons, as in the population at large.

Each of these findings has applicability for policies and programs for elderly mentally retarded persons. For example, retirement options could include a shift from scheduled or fixed day program participation to less regular, more individually tailored day program schedules. Part-time scheduling could be available for persons wanting to continue day program participation but at a less intense level. Further, the acknowledgement that the lifespan development of a mentally retarded person includes a period of time associated with the pursuit of leisure interests and relaxation may become more widely accepted. As the number of years spent in retirement increases for the general population, this option may be viewed as more acceptable for elders with mental retardation.

The retirement of mentally retarded persons from various types of day programs obviously opens new opportunities for other mentally retarded persons to enter those positions (or "slots"). The lack of an adequate number of slots is a major problem across the country in meeting the needs of persons not currently in the service system who are now, as adults, seeking meaningful day placements outside their family homes.

Finally, studies of the factors affecting the decision to retire for the nonretarded elderly population highlight the importance of personal expectations and attitudes, health status, and financial security. Given the general poverty of the population with mental retardation, economic concerns are unlikely to play as pivotal a role in the decisionmaking process regarding retirement for this group.

Further, it may well be that if a retarded person retires, the choice has been exercised by someone other than the retiree. The decision to retire for a person with mental retardation generally must be sanctioned or agreed to by professionals charged with the care of the individual. These professionals may also decide (along with the retiree) what the individual's activity options are during retirement. State or federal regulations regarding the day program requirements of residents of licensed residential programs often preclude consideration of as broad a range of retirement-oriented leisure and recreational activities as is typically available to the nonretarded elder. Thus, retirement decisions for or by mentally retarded individuals are rarely made without considerable

input from professionals or without consideration of regulatory requirements. These factors serve to constrain the freedom of choice that is
theoretically available to nonretarded elders when they retire.

RESULTS FROM THE
NATIONAL SURVEY

The National Survey gathered information about retirement options
for persons with mental retardation in three areas. First, information was
collected about retirement options currently existing in community-based
day programs for elderly mentally retarded persons. Such programs
include all of the community-based day program types discussed in
Chapter 6 except for vocational day activity programs.

Second, information was collected from institutionally based residential programs on whether clients had the option to retire from their day
programs. Information was also collected on the extent to which
institutionalized residents exercised the option to retire and the types of
activities in which retired residents participated. These results were
presented in Chapter 7.

Third, information on the prevalence of retirement options among
community-based residential programs serving elderly mentally retarded
persons was collected. Qualitative information was also collected from
these programs regarding the types of retirement policies that have been
developed and the programmatic impacts of retired residents on the
programs. These findings are presented in this chapter.

Thus, the purpose of this chapter is to describe the extent to which
retirement is a programmatic option within the community-based
residential programs that participated in the National Survey. The chapter
also examines salient differences between community-based residential
programs that had retirement options and those that did not.

PREVALENCE OF RETIREMENT
OPTIONS WITHIN
COMMUNITY-BASED
RESIDENTIAL PROGRAMS

Of the 186 community-based residential programs, slightly less than
half (43.4%) reported availability of a retirement option for residents.
Between one-third and one-half of the programs within each of the six
community-based residential types reported that their residents had the
option to retire (see Table 10-1). While the differences were not statistically
significant, group homes were the least likely to have such an option (38%

TABLE 10-1

Percentage of Community-Based Residential Programs with
Retirement Option for Residents ($N = 182$)

TYPE OF PROGRAM	PERCENT WITH RETIREMENT OPTION
Foster homes	44.0
Group homes	38.0
Group homes with nurses	42.3
ICFs/MR	45.2
Apartment programs	47.4
Mixed residential programs	50.0

of the programs), and mixed residential programs were the most likely to have such an option (50% of the programs).

Interestingly, virtually all programs with retirement options described their policy as based on the resident's preference for retirement. In several programs, for example, the resident's preference was conveyed to the members of an interdisciplinary team that met to establish the resident's formal program requirements. The resident was then allowed either to stay at home during the day or to participate in a generic senior center on a part-time basis. Some of the programs noted that at a specific age (i.e., age 55, 62, or 65), pre-planned discussions were held with the resident regarding his or her preference for either continued full-time, part-time, or no involvement with the current day program.

Respondents for community-based residential programs that claimed to have retirement options were asked if any residents in fact exercised this option. Less than half of the foster homes (40%), group homes (44.4%), group homes with nurses (44.5%), and apartment programs (44.4%) that permitted residents to retire had any retired residents. In contrast, two-thirds (68.4%) of the ICFs/MR and almost all (87.5%) of the mixed residential programs with retirement options had residents who were retired.

It was surprising that less than one-third of the respondents for residential programs with retirement options reported that having retired residents had an impact on their staffing (32.5%) for the program. One noted that its staff had simply adjusted their working hours to conform to the residents' schedule that included more in-home hours during the day. Another respondent said it had increased the number of hours spent by its activities coordinator per week. One respondent said that it was necessary to employ an additional day staff person for the days when the semi-retired residents remained at home.

Only a few programs with a retirement option (10.3%) reported that their funding was affected by having retired residents. One respondent noted that "it costs more to provide activities for clients staying at home."

Offering alternative activities for retired residents was cited as a problematic issue by only about a quarter (28.9%) of the respondents for programs with retired residents. Several respondents noted that linkages with generic senior centers had been sought to provide options for residents who were retired. Other respondents noted that conforming to state regulations regarding day program activities for residents (in terms of hours per day of programming) was particularly difficult with retired or semi-retired clients. Another program's respondent noted that having retired residents "changed the pace of the house."

It was not the norm, however, for community-based residential programs with a retirement option to have *all* of their residents retire. For those programs with retired residents, only mixed residential programs had on an average more than a third of their residents who were retired (37.5% of the residents). The ICF/MR and apartment program types had the next largest average percentage of residents who were retired (29.9% and 25.0%, respectively). Less than a fifth of the residents in foster homes (18.3%), group homes (16.7%), or group homes with nurses (12.3%) that permitted residents to retire were, in fact, retired. These findings suggest that the option to retire will be differentially utilized by residents. If as described by respondents the choice of retirement is given to the individual, a substantial number of elderly mentally retarded persons seem to choose to continue their participation in day programs beyond the time at which they could modify their day program activity or retire.

CHARACTERISTICS OF
PROGRAMS WITH RETIREMENT
OPTIONS

It was hypothesized that residential programs that offered retirement options differed with respect to their organizational, programmatic, or served population characteristics from programs that did not have such policies or options. In order to test this hypothesis, a series of comparisons were made among the 103 community-based residential programs with retirement options and the 79 programs without the option. The organizational, programmatic and client character' istics variables described in Chapters 5 and 6 were used in these analyses.

Table 10-2 presents the 10 variables for which significant differences were found between the two groups of residential programs. Programs with retirement options were more likely to have been expressly created to serve the elderly mentally retarded population. These programs were less likely to have physicians, psychologists, or social workers as part of the

TABLE 10-2

Differences Between Community-Based Residential Programs with and without a Retirement Option ($N = 182$)

VARIABLE	PROGRAM HAS NO RETIREMENT OPTION ($n = 103$)	PROGRAM HAS RETIREMENT OPTION ($n = 79$)	t
1. Program was created to serve EMR residents	.38	.56	-2.28^*
2. Program has physician on staff	.11	.01	2.84^{**}
3. Program has psychologist on staff	.24	.05	3.91^{***}
4. Program has social worker on staff	.40	.23	2.46^{**}
5. Percent of residents 22–50 years old	15	10	2.02^*
6. Percent of EMR residents severely/profoundly retarded	28	19	1.95^*
7. Percent of EMR residents judged in excellent health	13	29	-3.12^{**}
8. Percent of EMR residents judged in good health	58	46	2.19^*
9. Percent of EMR residents attending senior citizen center	4	12	-2.05^*
10. Percent of EMR residents attending day activity program	21	11	2.22^*

$^* = p<.05.$ $^{**} = p<.01.$ $^{***} = p<.001.$

core staff. These programs were also less likely to serve mentally retarded persons under age 50 and severely or profoundly retarded elders, but more likely to serve elderly mentally retarded persons who were described as being in excellent health given their age and level of disabilities. Further, programs with retirement options were more likely to have residents participating in generic senior centers (as expected), but less likely to have mentally retarded persons participating in day activity programs.

These results suggest that, organizationally and programmatically, programs with retirement options are somewhat different from programs without retirement options. Programs with retirement options were often consciously designed to meet the needs of elderly mentally retarded persons, whereas programs without retirement options were often those whose residents were simply aging in place. The characteristics of the elderly mentally retarded persons served in the former type of program also differed in some important respects from the characteristics of these in the latter group. For example, programs with retirement options tended to serve a healthier, less severely cognitively impaired group. As was discussed in Chapter 9, these are the types of elders with mental retardation who were found to be easier to integrate into generic senior centers.

CHARACTERISTICS OF
PROGRAMS WITH
RETIRED RESIDENTS

As noted earlier, simply having a retirement option did not mean that a program actually had residents who were retired. In order to identify organizational, programmatic, and client characteristics associated with programs having retired residents, a comparative analysis was conducted between these programs and those without retired residents. Again, the variables described in Chapters 5 and 6 were utilized to compare the 34 programs with retirement options but no retired residents with the 41 programs with retirement options and retired residents. Table 10-3 presents the variables for which significant differences were found.

Programs with retired residents were less likely to be located in a multiprogram agency and less likely to have received special funds for serving elders. These programs were also less likely to employ teachers and to provide psychological services to elderly mentally retarded residents, but more likely to offer transportation services. With respect to client characteristics, these programs had lower percentages of their

TABLE 10-3

Differences Between Community-Based Residential Programs with a
Retirement Option that Have Retired Residents
and that Do Not Have Retired Residents ($N = 75$)

VARIABLE	PROGRAM HAS NO RETIRED RESIDENTS ($n = 34$)	PROGRAM HAS NO RETIRED RESIDENTS ($n = 41$)	t
1. Multiprogram sponsoring agency	.94	.78	2.08*
2. Program received special funds	.35	.09	2.67**
3. Program has teachers on staff	.18	.02	2.15*
4. Program provides psychological services to EMR residents	.35	.15	2.12*
5. Program provides transportation for EMR residents	.68	.95	−3.11**
6. Percent of residents aged 51–54	11	5	1.96*
7. Percent of residents aged 55–60	29	15	2.67**
8. Age of oldest resident (years)	70.00	77.80	−4.09***
9. Percent of EMR who are female	55	38	2.02*
10. Percent of EMR residents at home with no formal program	4	28	−3.80***

$* = p<.05.$ $** = p<.01.$ $*** = p<.001.$

residents who were in the 51–54 and 55–60 age groups. The mean age of their oldest resident was significantly higher than for programs without retired residents. The percentage of elderly females among the total residential group was also lower in the programs with retired residents. Finally, these programs had a higher percentage of residents who remained at home with no formal program than did programs without retired residents (as expected).

These findings suggest that programs with retired residents differed from programs without retired residents (even though both groups in this analysis had retirement options) with respect to the characteristics of their residents. These programs tended to serve an older group of residents with a higher percentage of males and to provide fewer psychological services to their residents. Organizational or programmatic characteristics were less likely to differentiate between the two groups of residential settings. This pattern is similar to that reported above in the analysis of characteristics of programs with and without retirement options.

CONCLUSIONS

According to national demographic trends, the proportion of an individual's life spent in retirement is increasing. Retirement has gained acceptability as a stage in life when the pursuit of leisure interest is sanctioned and as a time when social expectations for individual productivity decline. It is particularly striking, therefore, that the issue of retirement for persons with mental retardation has received relatively scant attention by policy makers and service planners. Despite the fact that at least 50% of the residents in participating programs in the National Survey were 55 years of age or over, less than half of the community-based residential programs offered residents the *option* to retire. Among those programs with a retirement option, less than a third of the residents, on the average, were in fact retired in any of the six community-based residential types.

Our findings were that, in general, client characteristics (such as being older, having a better reported health status, being less severely retarded, and being male) were stronger correlates of whether a residential program had a retirement option or had retired clients than were organizational or programmatic characteristics. Further, we found that simply having a retirement option did not mean that the program served retired clients exclusively. We were encouraged by these general patterns, which suggest that programs develop retirement policies based on the character of the population they serve rather than as a matter of organizational or programmatic principle. Thus, to some extent the age-specialized programs participating in the National Survey did provide individualized choices to their residents regarding retirement opportunities.

As described in Chapters 6, 7, 8, and 9, retirement options do exist within the day program components of many community and institution-ally based service systems. The program models we have described are characterized by their diversity in structure, organizational features, and programmatic emphasis. Assuming that there will be continued develop-ment of alternative day programs for mentally retarded seniors as the size of this group grows, it can be anticipated that the number of residential programs supporting residents' retirement will increase as well.

Chapter 11

Extending the Continuum
Agenda for Research, Service, and Policy Development

In this monograph, we have described specialized programs that have extended the continuum of services to meet the needs of mentally retarded persons once they have reached old age. The purpose of this chapter is to distill key findings from the National Survey and to present our assessment of the major research, service, and policy issues that comprise the agenda for continued knowledge and program development in this area.

KEY FINDINGS

Detailed information on the 529 community and institutionally based residential and day programs that participated in the National Survey was presented in Chapters 5 through 8. Our analyses yielded both similarities and differences among the programs surveyed. In the sections that follow, we present some general summary findings regarding significant organizational, programmatic, and client characteristics of these specialized programs.

Organizational Characteristics

One of the most striking findings of the National Survey was the rapid increase in the number of programs for elderly mentally retarded persons that began operation during the last 10 years. While there were a few programs that served older mentally retarded clients prior to that time, the majority of the programs in the National Survey were of relatively recent origin.

Our findings further indicated that the programs for elderly mentally retarded persons were stable and structurally well integrated into the pre-existing service delivery system. We base this conclusion on four distinct findings. First, as shown in Chapter 4, the specialized programs serving elderly mentally retarded persons were located across the country in both institutionally and community-based service systems. Further, we found a rich variety of program models within both the day and residential service components of these systems. This level of geographic and programmatic diversity illustrated the infusion of such programs within the major components of the mental retardation service system.

Second, these programs were sponsored by all types of agencies—private for-profit, private nonprofit, proprietary, and state-operated providers. Most were multiprogram agencies. While the majority of the programs were sponsored by agencies in the mental retardation service system, we also found programs that were sponsored by agencies within the aging network of services. Thus, there was a remarkable degree of diversity among the types of agencies sponsoring specialized programs for elderly mentally retarded persons.

Third, we found a fairly even split between the prevalence of specially created programs and programs that had evolved into the care of elderly mentally retarded persons. This suggests two strengths of the mental retardation system. On the one hand, it suggests that the system is capable of responding to new service needs within its pre-existing program models. On the other hand, it suggests that the system is capable of generating new program types to meet newly recognized needs. Further, the created programs were not, in general, demonstration projects, which typically have uncertain long term stability. Rather, we found that the created programs in the National Survey included few demonstration projects and instead were more likely to have been supported by traditional sources of funds and sponsored by multiprogram agencies.

A fourth indication of the stability of programs for elderly mentally retarded persons was that every program in the National Survey expected to continue to serve this population in the future. When asked what changes were anticipated during the coming year, not one program indicated that it expected to be closed or that it would cease serving elderly mentally retarded persons.

These findings indicated an impressive degree of structural and programmatic integration and stability of specialized programs for elderly mentally retarded clients within the existing mental retardation service delivery system. This was an important conclusion because the number of elderly mentally retarded persons is predicted to increase dramatically in the coming years (Lubin & Kiely, 1985). It further demonstrated that the continuum of services has been extended to meet the needs of mentally retarded persons across the full life cycle.

Programmatic Characteristics

Our analyses of the community-based residential and day programs yielded two distinct typologies. The residential program typology may be characterized by its similarity in both diversity and structure to traditional residential typologies within the mental retardation service system. Regarding diversity, we identified residential programs that were service rich and those that were service poor. We further found residential programs that had a wide variety of professional staff and those that were primarily operated by nonprofessionals. These differences mirrored the diversity in service and staff capabilities known to exist within the general community-based residential system for persons with mental retardation.

There was also a remarkable degree of structural similarity between the residential programs that participated in the National Survey and those that serve younger mentally retarded adults. There was only one residential program type that was newly identified in our typology: the group home with nurses model (see Chapter 5). This program model was an important modification of the most prevalent type of community residence. The addition of a nurse to the core staff of a group home was clearly an adaptive response to the health needs of the residents served in such programs.

Our basic conclusion was that the community-based residential component of the service system had demonstrated its elasticity to meet the needs of various types of clients—including elderly mentally retarded persons. This important finding suggests that as mentally retarded persons age, their residential placements need not necessarily change. Given the stress associated with residential change at any age, but particularly for older persons (Heller, 1985; Tobin & Lieberman, 1976), the capacity of the residential setting to remain stable over time seemed to us to be an important programmatic characteristic.

In contrast with the residential typology, we found that there has been a remarkable degree of innovation within the community-based day program service sector. The types of community-based day programs that emerged from our analyses did not fit neatly into any of the day program typologies that had been presented in the literature and that were summarized in Chapter 6. Specialized day programs for elderly mentally retarded persons ranged from vocationally oriented, full-time programs to part-time leisure and outreach programs. Some programs maintained staffing ratios comparable to those in day programs for younger mentally retarded adults. Others, particularly the leisure and outreach programs, had fewer staff per client. These programmatic differences reflected the variability in the cognitive abilities of clients, the goals of the programs, and the programs' resources. In summary, the community-based day program typology displayed a substantial level of adaptability and innovation by the agencies that developed these options.

We were surprised that no distinct typologies emerged from our analyses of residential and day programs located in institutional settings.

While institutionally based residential and day programs differed from each other in organizational, programmatic, and client characteristics, the programs surveyed *within* the residential and *within* the day program sectors were comparatively homogeneous. We attributed these findings to the powerful influence of the federal regulations that govern institutions receiving Medicaid funds. These regulations may have curbed the institution's capacity to provide a range of different types of programs for the elderly within the institution. The regulations did not, however, seem to curb the institutions' capacity to develop specialized programs, as there were many that participated in the National Survey (nearly 40% of the total sample of programs).

We were also surprised at the unexpectedly high rate at which institutionally based programs accessed community-based generic senior centers on behalf of their clients. Many professionals have urged increased integration of elderly mentally retarded persons with the general elderly population through their joint utilization of senior centers (Janicki, Knox, & Jacobson, 1985). It is encouraging that the most segregated service system for mentally retarded persons—the institution—has had considerable success in integrating mentally retarded seniors with the nonretarded elderly population.

There were several programmatic commonalities among the institutionally and community-based residential and day programs. First, the majority of the programs (irrespective of location or type) served both younger (under age 55) and older (age 55 and above) mentally retarded persons. Thus, while the use of a specific age criterion is important for determining program eligibility for some purposes (such as in programs funded through the Older Americans Act or for benefits under the Social Security Administration) and for defining a population for study, most of the programs included in the National Survey were not stringent in their use of an age-based eligibility criterion.

Second, programs that received Medicaid funding (such as the community-based ICFs/MR and many institutionally based programs), as well as programs governed by state regulations that have adopted the active treatment standards of Medicaid regulations, faced particular problems in serving elderly mentally retarded persons. Specifically, respondents noted that there was a need to "creatively circumvent" regulations that required a participant to receive 6 hours a day of active treatment unless the participant received a medically based waiver. The perceived need to circumvent the regulations was based on the declining motivation or capacity of an elder to continue his or her participation in a day program that was either viewed as no longer appropriate (especially if the program was oriented toward vocational skills training) or as requiring more stamina and regularity of participation than the elder could sustain. For these persons, the need to allow for either flexibly scheduled participation in pre-existing day programs or the development of special programs primarily oriented toward recreational and leisure time pursuits was particularly acute.

Finally, a considerable amount of discomfort was expressed by respondents across all types of programs regarding the fact that for many elderly mentally retarded persons, *maintenance* rather than *development* of skills may be the most appropriate goal. This discomfort reflected the influence of the developmental model on the goals of services within the mental retardation system. The developmental model postulates that all individuals are capable of lifelong learning and, further, that individuals vary primarily in terms of their rate of learning, not in their capacity for learning (MacMillan, 1982). Consistent with this philosophy, individualized service plans typically specify the programs or services needed for clients to achieve new skills—not to maintain existing skills. In contrast, gerontologists have demonstrated that the maintenance of skills is an appropriate goal for many persons who are aging, because without the specified services many elders would experience a loss of skills (Granger, Seltzer, & Fishbein, 1987; House & Robbins, 1983).

Despite the reality of the consequences of the aging process, at the present time the standards governing the development of individualized service plans for elderly mentally retarded persons may constrain professionals' ability to specify maintenance of skills as a legitimate goal. According to many respondents for programs in the National Survey, the programmatic consequences of current standards were that either programs had to be described as skill building programs despite the fact that they were not in fact so oriented, or that "creative writing" was required to mask the fact that maintenance of skills was the real goal for some individuals.

Client Characteristics

The programs that participated in the National Survey served a heterogeneous group of elderly mentally retarded persons. These programs varied with respect to the age range of clients served, their levels of retardation, and their reported health status. This variability is consistent with past research that has established that elders with mental retardation are not uniform in their characteristics (Janicki & MacEachron, 1984; Krauss & Seltzer, 1986). However, it also reflects the fact the programs have not restricted their services to particularly frail, particularly old, or particularly cognitively impaired individuals from the larger population of elders with mental retardation. This can clearly be seen as a strength of the programmatic offerings currently available to this population.

Further, client characteristics were found to be important correlates of a number of programmatic and policy-relevant outcomes. For example, client characteristics were correlated with the provision of retirement options within community-based residential programs, with the receptivity of generic senior centers staff and nonretarded elders towards elderly mentally retarded persons, and with the level of community participation achieved by community-based day programs. These findings suggest that programmatic and policy goals must be differentially articulated for each of the various types of elderly mentally retarded persons. It may not be reasonable, for example, to assume that *all* elderly mentally retarded persons are good candidates for retirement or for receiving services through the generic aging network's programs.

AGENDA FOR RESEARCH, SERVICE, AND POLICY DEVELOPMENT

The preceding discussion of some of the key findings of the National Survey contains many implications for needed research, service, and policy development. The service system for elderly mentally retarded persons is in an early stage of development. The degree of interest in and commitment to the continued expansion and refinement of program models by respondents to the National Survey was impressive. Based on their reports, experiences, and recommendations, we have formulated a range of agenda items that will hopefully make a contribution to the specification of well grounded and programmatically effective service for elderly mentally retarded persons. The research, service, and policy agenda items are summarized in this section.

Research Agenda

While some research has been conducted on aging and mental retardation during the past ten years, from a scientific perspective, rigorous studies are needed in a number of areas. Among these are the following.

Determination of the size and age distribution of the elderly population with mental retardation.

As we discussed in Chapter 2, valid prevalence estimates of the population of elders with mental retardation are not currently available.

Commonly used prevalence estimates are often based on untested or unverified assumptions about the chronological onset of old age for this population, the current life expectancy of mentally retarded persons, and the durability of the diagnosis of mental retardation throughout the life cycle. These estimates are also typically based on state registries of current service recipients. Such estimates are inherently conservative, as many elders with mental retardation are not known to the formal service delivery system (Krauss, 1986). Future research on elderly mentally retarded persons will be strengthened by the resolution of these definitional, epidemiological, and methodological issues.

Evaluation of the types of programs that are most effective in meeting the needs of elderly mentally retarded persons.

The National Survey provided descriptive accounts of a series of program prototypes. We made no attempt to evaluate the relative effectiveness of these program models. However, the extent of between-model diversity that characterized the community-based residential and day program typologies argues for the need to study their differential effectiveness for different subgroups of elders with mental retardation. The person-environment fit concept (Landesman & Butterfield, 1987; Landesman-Dwyer, 1984) is particularly important in light of the heterogeneity of the population of elders with mental retardation. Comparative studies of the effects of the various program types on specific subgroups of elderly mentally retarded persons are needed. This information will further our understanding of the best methods of meeting the different service needs of this heterogeneous and vulnerable population.

Examination of the age-related changes in health, cognitive abilities and functional status of elders with mental retardation.

The development of the full range of services for elderly mentally retarded persons is dependent on an understanding of the pattern of expected changes associated with the aging process. Gerontological researchers have conducted studies of large samples of adults spanning several decades (Busse & Maddox, 1985, for example) in order to generate a scientific understanding of normative age-related trends. Comparable longitudinal research is needed to provide an understanding of these trends for elders with mental retardation. However, most of the available research on this population has used cross-sectional research designs (M. Seltzer, 1985). Thus, cohort effects, which are very substantial in this population, cannot be separated out from the effects of aging.

In addition to generating knowledge about age-related trends and differences, longitudinal research will enable the field to more precisely define *elderly* in the population with mental retardation. Currently, there is no consensus among researchers, policy analysts, or service providers as to what, if any, chronological age should define the onset of old age. Because we have a very imprecise understanding of the pattern of decline for mentally retarded persons as they age, we have no scientific basis for chronologically defining the beginning of this stage of life. Longitudinal research would make an important contribution to this definitional issue.

Assessment of the impacts of various service options on personal satisfaction and quality of life of elderly mentally retarded persons.

Research on the general elderly population has suggested that there may be an inverse correlation between life satisfaction and morbidity (Larson, 1978). This relationship remains virtually unexplored in mentally retarded elders and warrants scientific study. While little is known about the factors that contribute to a high level of life satisfaction and quality of life for mentally retarded elders, the need to examine these issues has been noted in the literature (Landesman, 1986). Among the factors to be examined are the impact of living in age-integrated versus age-segregated housing, of continuing to participate in work activities or active treatment programs versus choosing to retire, and of using generic senior citizens programs versus remaining in specialized programs for elderly mentally retarded persons.

Further, there is a need to examine the psychological stresses experienced by elderly mentally retarded persons as they age and deal with the loss of family and friends, their own increasing frailty, and their increasing number of health impairments (G. Seltzer, 1985). These issues were identified by respondents in the National Survey as of central importance to an understanding of the quality of life of elderly service recipients and thus are in need of substantial examination in future research.

Service Development Agenda

The National Survey documented the geometric rate of increase in the number of specialized programs for elderly mentally retarded persons that have begun during the past 10 years. There is clearly an increased recognition by service providers of the need to serve elderly mentally retarded persons and a heightened commitment to extending the continuum of services for this purpose. In this context, a number of challenges currently face the mental retardation service system. Among these challenges are the following.

Assessment of the feasibility of each of the three service options.

Three service options were identified in Chapter 1: the age-integration option, in which elderly mentally retarded persons are served in programs designed for younger retarded persons; the generic services integration option, in which elderly mentally retarded persons are served in programs designed for nonretarded elderly persons; and the specialized service option, such as the programs included in the National Survey. These three options should be assessed to determine their relative efficacy for different types of clients. The differential impact of serving elderly mentally retarded persons in age-integrated versus age-specialized programs should be examined in order to identify the optimal mix of service options for this client group. Further, the administrative feasibility of the three service patterns warrants critical examination.

Prioritization of service goals for elderly mentally retarded persons.

The literature notes a wide variety of goals that should be considered in providing services to elderly mentally retarded persons (Janicki et al., 1985). These goals include:
- to provide clients with continuity and stability of home life and interpersonal relationships,
- to offer clients new opportunities for age-appropriate retirement activities,
- to enable clients to develop new skills as they age,
- to assist clients to maintain the skills they have already acquired,
- to prevent or delay placement in a nursing home or an institution.

As services develop and become more differentiated, it becomes possible to consider how each of these goals is differentially applicable to each elder with mental retardation. It is important for service providers to recognize that in choosing to meet some of these goals, others might not be met. For example, ensuring continuity of an individual's own residence might not be conducive to offering new opportunities to him or her for age-appropriate retirement activities. Service providers must be prepared to prioritize these and other related goals for each elder with mental retardation and to be ready to set aside seemingly desirable goals that may conflict with more important needs of the individual.

*Exploration of the meaning of retirement and personal choice in the
lifestyles of elderly mentally retarded persons.*

Many planners and service providers have articulated the need for
active retirement programs. These programs are often defined by their
substitution of leisure and recreational activities for vocational activities.
Further, many professionals believe that elderly mentally retarded
persons should choose the particular retirement activities in which they
will participate. In order to make a rational choice, a person must have an
understanding of and an appreciation for the range of possible activities
from which to choose. It may be worthwhile to question whether this
expectation can be introduced for the first time once an individual has
reached old age. Rather, the development of personal preferences is a
lifelong process. When a mentally retarded elder reaches the point of
expressing personal preferences, he or she becomes an excellent candidate
for active retirement.

*Development of a plan for outreach to currently unserved elderly
mentally retarded persons.*

There are many elderly mentally retarded persons—perhaps 40% of
this population—who are not known to receive formal services from the
mental retardation service system. Such persons presumably are
supported and cared for by relatives. Currently, it is common for such
individuals to be identified by the service system in the midst of a crisis,
such as the death or impairment of a parent or other relative. Service
providers must develop community-based residential models that can
provide a safety net for the dependent retarded family member in such
circumstances. In a related vein, service providers must be as supportive
as possible to involved family members in order to maximize their capacity
to continue to provide support for aging mentally retarded relatives as
they themselves age (Dobrof, 1985).

Policy Agenda

At the present time, programs and services for elderly mentally
retarded persons are proliferating on a grassroots level. However, they are
developing generally without the benefit of federal or state policies that
could provide a context for their development. A series of federal and
state level policy issues have emerged that warrant immediate attention.
These include the following.

Development of a plan for interagency collaboration between the mental retardation service system and the aging network.

Elderly mentally retarded persons are eligible for the services and programs provided by two service delivery sectors: mental retardation and aging. Janicki, Ackerman, and Jacobson (1985), in a nationwide study, found that the frequency of formal interagency coordination between these two service sectors was very low. Indeed, when we contacted each of the 50 state units on aging for the National Survey, most referred us to their counterparts in the mental retardation state agencies (see Chapter 3). Thus, at the present time administrative responsibility for elders with mental retardation is lodged primarily within the mental retardation service system.

There has been a great deal of interest expressed in exploring the resources, program models, and service packages available to the general elderly population and the applicability of these resources to mentally retarded elders. For example, adult day care centers, senior citizens programs, homemaking services, and chore services are routinely utilized by the general elderly population when they are frail or infirm (Lowy, 1985a). While mentally retarded elders may be eligible for these resources, we have little information regarding the likely organizational impact of sharing such resources on the two service sectors. Policy analysis is needed to assess the feasibility and desirability of more intensive interagency collaboration and resource allocation for the population of elders with mental retardation.

Modification of programmatic regulations to respond to the retirement needs of elders with mental retardation.

In many states the underlying philosophy of regulations governing programs for mentally retarded persons of all ages is *habilitation* (Seltzer, Sherwood, & Litchfield, 1982). This is operationalized through a variety of programmatic mechanisms emphasizing *active treatment* (Manfredini & Smith, in press). The field has devoted insufficient attention to developing an operational definition of habilitation for elders with mental retardation. One impact of the current view on active treatment is that by virtue of living in a state licensed facility, mentally retarded elders may be precluded from retiring. While the results of the National Survey indicate that many programs have found ways either to circumvent these regulations or to have the regulations waived, it is important that clear policies regarding retirement of mentally retarded persons be developed. In this respect, more studies are needed that compare the impact of continued imposition of active treatment requirements with the impact of waiving such requirements for reasons other than medical limitations. These analyses and studies will provide an indication of how the goal of habilitation should be operationalized for elders with mental retardation.

Increased budgetary allocations for specialized programs serving elderly mentally retarded persons.

In general, the provision of services to elderly individuals may be more expensive than provision of similar services to younger adults. For example, there may be an increased need for transportation services for the elderly, an increased need to modify the physical environment, and an increased need for medical, nursing, and nutritional consultation. The fiscal implications of meeting the general service needs of elderly mentally retarded persons have not been directly addressed by service planners or policy analysts.

In this context, the addition of a nurse to the staff of a group home represents an important modification of the traditional group home model that was identified in the National Survey. However, the inclusion of a nursing position in the staffing pattern of a community-based residential program presumably results in increased personnel costs. Similarly, specialized residential programs with retirement options may have to supplement their staffing plans and budgets in order to provide daytime staffing coverage (see Chapter 10). While the National Survey did not provide a budgetary analysis of these and other programmatic components, state agencies may be faced with the need to offer higher levels of funding to specialized programs for elderly mentally retarded persons than to age-integrated programs and services.

Provision of state-level incentives for the development of innovative programs for elderly mentally retarded persons.

The day and residential program typologies that emerged from the National Survey attest to the diversity of specialized programs for elderly mentally retarded persons. Nevertheless, it is important to refrain from viewing these program types as the only or necessarily the best ways to serve the population of elders with mental retardation. State agencies must be sure to continue to build diversity into services for mentally retarded elders. We highlighted three types of service options earlier—the age-integration option, the generic services integration option, and the specialized services option. While each has merit, policy and program analysts should be committed to the continued development and evaluation of new service models for this population.

CONCLUSIONS

The National Survey uncovered an unexpected large number of specialized residential and day programs for elderly mentally retarded persons. In both the institutional and the community-based service sectors, the range of programmatic innovations developed to serve this group was remarkable. While many of the programs had evolved into the care of elderly mentally retarded persons, an equal number were intentionally created for this purpose. Thus, the service delivery system has demonstrated both elasticity and planned responsiveness to new needs.

Clearly the experiences of these pioneering programs suggest that new challenges are presented in serving elderly mentally retarded persons. We have offered some suggestions regarding research, service, and policy agenda that warrant professional attention. Continued innovation and extension of the continuum of services for elderly mentally retarded persons will be required as the size of this group grows and as the lessons from these initial programmatic efforts are systematically and rigorously investigated.

References

Anderson, R. (1984). *Planning a program for older developmentally disabled clients*. McCook, NE: Region II Services for the Handicapped.

Anglin, B. (1981). *They never asked for help: A study on the needs of elderly retarded people in Metro Toronto*. Ontario: Belsten Publishing.

Atchley, R.C. (1982). Retirement as a social institution. *Annual Review of Sociology, 8*, 263–287.

Axel, H., & Brotman, H.B. (1982). Demographics of the mature work force. In D. Bauer (Ed.) *Significant segment—Employment and training of the mature worker: A resource manual.* (pp. 14–42). Washington, D.C.: National Council on the Aging, Inc.

Bailey, P.P. (1983). Testimony before U.S. Senate Special Committee on Aging. May 25.

Baird, P.A., & Sadovnick, A.D. (1985). Mental retardation in over half-a-million consecutive livebirths: An epidemiological study. *American Journal of Mental Deficiency, 89*, 323–330.

Baker, B.L., Seltzer, G.B., & Seltzer, M.M. (1977). *As close as possible: Community residences for retarded adults*. Boston: Little, Brown & Co.

Ball, R.M. (1983). Testimony before U.S. Senate Special Committee on Aging. May 25.

Barfield, R.E., & Morgan, J.N. (1969). *Early retirement: The decision and the experience*. Ann Arbor: The University of Michigan.

Baroff, G.S. (1982). Predicting the prevalence of mental retardation in individual catchment areas. *Mental Retardation, 20*, 133–135.

Berkson, G., & Romer, D. (1980). Social ecology of supervised communal facilities for mentally disabled adults: I. Introduction. *American Journal of Mental Deficiency, 85*, 219–228.

Best-Sigford, B., Bruininks, R.H., Lakin, L.C., Hill, B.K., & Heal, L.W. (1982). Resident release patterns in a national sample of public residential facilities. *American Journal of Mental Deficiency, 87*, 130–140.

Birren, J.E. (1959). Principles of research on aging. In J.E. Birren (Ed.), *Handbook of aging in the individual.* (pp. 3–42). Chicago: University of Chicago Press.

Boggs, E., Lakin, K.C., & Clauser, S. (1985). Medicaid coverage of residential services. In K.C. Lakin, B. Hill, & R.H. Bruininks (Eds.), *An analysis of medicaid: Intermediate care facility for the mentally retarded (ICF/MR) program* (pp. 1-1 to 1-78). Minneapolis: University of Minnesota, Department of Educational Psychology.

Branch, L.G. (1987). Continuing care retirement communities: Self-insuring for long-term care. *The Gerontologist, 27*, 4–8.

Brody, E. (1979). Aged parents and aging children. In P.K. Ragan (Ed.), *Aging parents.* (pp. 267–287). Los Angeles: University of Southern California Press.

Brody, E.M. (1985). Parent care as a normative family stress. *The Gerontologist, 25*, 19–29.

Brooks, D.N. Wooley, A., & Kanjilal, G.C. (1972). Hearing loss and middle ear disorders in patients with Down's (Mongolism). *Journal of Mental Deficiency Research, 16*, 21–29.

Busse, E.W., & Maddox, G.L. (1985). *The Duke longitudinal studies of normal aging 1955–1980: Overview of history, design, and findings*. New York: Springer.

Butler, E.L. (Ed.) (1976). *A consultation-conference on the gerontological aspects of mental retardation*. Mississippi Department of Mental Health and Mississippi Council on Aging.

Butler, E.W., & Bjaanes, A.T. (1977). A typology of community care facilities and differential normalization outcomes. In P. Mittler (Ed.), *Research to practice in mental retardation. Vol. I. Care and intervention.* (pp. 337–347). Baltimore: University Park Press.

Callahan, J., & Wallack, S. (Eds.) (1981). *Reforming the long-term-care system*. Lexington, MA: Lexington Books.

Callison, D.A., Armstrong, H.F., Elam, L., Cannon, R.L., Paisley, C.M., & Himwich, H. (1971). The effects of aging on schizophrenic and mentally defective patients: Visual, auditory, and grip strength measurements. *Journal of Gerontology, 26,* 137–145.

Campbell, V.A., & Bailey, C.J. (1984). Comparison of methods for classifying community residential settings for mentally retarded individuals. *American Journal of Mental Deficiency, 89,* 44–49.

Cantor, M.H. (1984). The family: A basic source of long-term care for the elderly. In P. Feinstein, M. Gornick, & J. Greenberg (Eds.), *Long-term care financing and delivery systems: Exploring some alternatives.* (pp. 107–112). Washington, D.C.: U.S. Department of Health and Human Services. (HCFA Publication No. 03174).

Carsrud, A.L., & Carsrud, K.B. (1983). *Effects of structured interaction on self and environmental awareness in geriatric mentally retarded* (Working Paper 83/84 - 4 31). Austin: University of Texas at Austin, Graduate School of Business.

Catapano, P.M., Levy, J.M., & Levy, P.H. (1985). Day activity and vocational program services. In M.P. Janicki and H.M. Wisniewski (Eds.), *Aging and developmental disabilities: Issues and approaches* (pp. 305–316). Baltimore: Paul H. Brookes.

Clark, R.L., & Barker, D.T. (1981). *Reversing the trend toward early retirement.* Washington, D.C.: American Enterprise Institute.

Cleveland, D.W., & Miller, N. (1977). Attitudes and life commitments of older siblings of mentally retarded adults: An exploratory study. *Mental Retardation, 15,* 38–41.

Cohen, D.L. (1980). Continuing-care communities for the elderly: Potential pitfalls and proposed legislation. *University of Pennsylvania Law Review, 128,* 883–936.

Congdon, D.M. (1983). *An alternative living program model for older developmentally disabled individuals.* Indianapolis: Indiana State Council on Developmental Disabilities.

Cotton, P.D., Purzycki, E., Cowart, C., & Merritt, F. (1983). *Changes in adaptive behavior of elderly mentally retarded as a function of community placement.* University of Southern Mississippi.

Cotton, P.D., Sison, G.F., & Starr, S. (1981). Comparing elderly mentally retarded and non-mentally retarded individuals: Who are they? What are their needs? *The Gerontologist, 21,,* 359–365.

Crnic, K.A., Friedrich, W.N., & Greenberg, M.T. (1983). Adaptation of families with mentally retarded children: A model of stress, coping, and family ecology. *American Journal of Mental Deficiency, 88,* 345–351.

DiGiovanni, L. (1978). The elderly retarded: A little-known group. *The Gerontologist, 18,* 262–266.

Dobrof, R. (1985). Some observations from the field of aging. In M.P. Janicki and H.M. Wisniewski (Eds.) *Aging and developmental disabilities: Issues and approaches.* (pp. 411–415). Baltimore: Paul H. Brookes.

Dubrow, A.L. (1967). *Are these the golden years? Dynamic programming in the rehabilitation of the aging.* Institute conducted by Northeastern University's Department of Rehabilitation and Special Education in cooperation with Rehabilitation Services Administration, Department of Health, Education, and Welfare, Dedham, MA.

Dy, E.B., Strain, P.S., Fullerton, A., & Stowitschek, J. (1981). Training institutionalized, elderly mentally retarded persons as intervention agents for socially isolated peers. *Analysis and Intervention in Developmental Disabilities, 1,* 199–215.

Dybwad, G. (1962). Administrative and legislative problems in the care of the adult and aged mental retardate. *American Journal of Mental Deficiency, 66,* 716–722.

Edgerton, R.B. (1967). *The cloak of competence: Stigma in the lives of the mentally retarded.* Berkeley: University of California Press.

Edgerton, R.B., Bollinger, M., & Herr, B. (1984). The cloak of competence: After two decades. *American Journal of Mental Deficiency, 88,* 345–351.

Eisdorfer, C. (1983). Conceptual models of aging: The challenge of a new frontier. *American Psychologist, 38,* 197–202.

Eyman, R.K., & Arndt, S. (1982). Life-span development of institutional and community-based mentally retarded residents. *American Journal of Mental Deficiency, 86,* 342–350.

Eyman, R., Grossman, H., Tarjan, G., & Miller, C. (1987). *Life expectancy and mental retardation: A longitudinal study in a state residential facility.* Washington, D.C.: American Association on Mental Deficiency.

Feinstein, P.H., Gornick, M., & Greenberg, J.N. (1984). The need for new approaches in long-term care. In P. Feinstein, M. Gornick, & J. Greenberg (Eds.), *Long-term care financing and delivery systems: Exploring some alternatives.* (pp. 7–12). Washington, D.C.: U.S. Department of Health and Human Services. (HCFA Publication No. 03174).

Gelwicks, L.E. (1984). Housing: The "where" in the continuum of care. In P. Feinstein, M. Gornick, & J. Greenberg (Eds.), *Long-term care financing and delivery systems: Exploring some alternatives.* (pp. 71–78). Washington, D.C.: U.S. Department of Health and Human Services. (HCFA Publication No. 03174).

Gollay, E., Freedman, R., Wyngaarden, M., & Kurtz, N.R. (1978). *Coming back: The community experiences of deinstitutionalized mentally retarded people.* Cambridge, MA: Abt Books.

Granger, C.V., Seltzer, G.B., & Fishbein, C. (1987). *Primary care of the functionally disabled: Assessment and management.* Philadelphia: Lippincott.

Greenberg, J.N., & Leutz, W.N. (1984). The social/health maintenance organization and its role in reforming the long-term care system. In P. Feinstein, M. Gornick, & J. Greenberg (Eds.). *Long-term care financing and delivery systems: Exploring some alternatives.* (pp. 57–65). Washington, D.C.: U.S. Department of Health and Human Services. (HCFA Publication No. 03174).

Grossman, H.J. (Ed.) (1983). *Classification in mental retardation.* Washington, D.C.: American Association on Mental Deficiency.

Halpern, A.S., Close, D.W., Nelson, D.J. (1986) *On my own: The impact of semi-independent living programs for adults with mental retardation.* Baltimore: Paul H. Brookes.

Hamilton, J., & Segal, R. (Eds.) (1975). *Proceedings of a consultation conference on the gerontological aspects of mental retardation.* Ann Arbor: University of Michigan.

Hauber, F.A., Bruininks, R.H., Hill, B.K., Lakin, K.C., & White, C.C. (1984). *National census of residential facilities: Fiscal year 1982.* Minneapolis: University of Minnesota, Department of Education Psychology.

Hauber, F.A., Bruininks, R.H., Hill, B.K., Lakin, K.C., Scheerenberger, R.C., & White, C.C. (1984). National census of residential facilities: A 1982 profile of facilities and residents. *American Journal of Mental Deficiency, 89,* 236–245.

Hauber, F.A., Rotegard, L.L., & Bruininks, R.H. (1985). Characteristics of residential services for older/elderly mentally retarded persons. In M.P. Janicki & H.M. Wisniewski (Eds.), *Aging and developmental disabilities: Issues and approaches.* (pp. 327–350) Baltimore: Paul H. Brookes.

Heller, T. (1985). Residential relocation and reactions of elderly mentally retarded persons. In M.P. Janicki and H.M. Wisniewski (Eds.), *Aging and developmental disabilities: Issues and approaches.* (pp. 379–390) Baltimore: Paul H. Brookes.

Hill, B.K., & Lakin, K.C. (1986). Classification of residential facilities for individuals with mental retardation. *Mental Retardation, 24,* 107–115.

Hooyman, N. (1983). Social support networks in services to the elderly. In J.K. Whittaker, J. Garbarino, and Associates (Eds.), *Social support networks: Informal helping in the human services.* (pp. 133–164). New York: Aldine Publishing Co.

House, J.S., & Robbins, C. (1983). Age, psychological stress, and health. In M.W. Riley, B.B. Hess, & K. Bond (Eds.), *Aging in society: Selected reviews of recent research.* (pp. 175–198). Hillsdale, NJ: Lawrence Erlbaum Associates.

Huttman, E.D. (1985). *Social services for the elderly.* New York: The Free Press.

Intagliata, J., & Doyle, N. (1984). Enhancing social support for parents of developmentally disabled children: Trading on interpersonal problem solving skills. *Mental Retardation, 22,* 4–11.

Jacobson, J.W., Sutton, M.S., & Janicki, M.P. (1985). Demography and characteristics of aging and aged mentally retarded persons. In M.P. Janicki and H.M. Wisniewski (Eds.), *Aging and developmental disabilities: Issues and approaches.* (pp. 115–142). Baltimore: Paul H. Brookes.

Janicki, M. Ackerman, L., & Jacobson, J. (1984). *Survey of state developmental disabilities and aging plans relative to states' older developmentally disabled population.* (Report #84-4).

Albany, New York: New York State Office of Mental Retardation and Developmental Disabilities.

Janicki, M.P., Ackerman, L., & Jacobson, J.W. (1985). State developmental disabilities/aging plans and planning for an older developmentally disabled population. *Mental Retardation, 23,* 297–301.

Janicki, M.P., & Jacobson, J.W. (1984a). *Behavioral abilities of older mentally retarded persons.* Paper presented at the 108th Annual Conference of the American Association on Mental Deficiency, Minneapolis, MN.

Janicki, M.P., & Jacobson, J.W. (1984b). *Health and support services for mentally retarded elders living in foster care and group homes.* Symposium conducted at the 37th Annual Scientific Meeting of the Gerontological Society of America, San Antonio, TX.

Janicki, M.P., & Jacobson, J.W. (1986a). *What do the data tell us about the aging and aged mentally retarded population.* Paper presented at the 110th Annual Conference of the American Association on Mental Deficiency, Denver, CO.

Janicki, M.P., & Jacobson, J.W. (1986b). Generational trends in sensory, physical, and behavioral abilities among older mentally retarded persons. *American Journal of Mental Deficiency, 90,* 490–500.

Janicki, M.P., Knox, L.A., & Jacobson, J.W. (1985). Planning for an older developmentally disabled population. In M.P. Janicki and H.M. Wisniewski (Eds.), *Aging and developmental disabilities: Issues and approaches.* (pp. 143–159). Baltimore: Paul H. Brookes.

Janicki, M.P., Krauss, M.W., & Seltzer, M.M. (Eds.) (in press). *Community residences for persons with developmental disabilities: Here to stay.* Baltimore: Paul H. Brookes.

Janicki, M.P., & MacEachron, A.E. (1984). Residential, health, and social service needs of elderly developmentally disabled persons. *The Gerontologist, 24,* 128–137.

Janicki, M.P., Otis, J.P., Puccio, P.S., Rettig, J.H., & Jacobson, J. (1985). Service needs among older developmentally disabled persons. In M.P. Janicki & H.M. Wisniewski (Eds.), *Aging and developmental disabilities: Issues and approaches.* (pp. 289–304). Baltimore: Paul H. Brookes.

Johnson, V.M., & Olsen, L.M. (1982). *A guide to alternative programming for older mentally retarded-developmentally disabled adults.* St. Louis, MO: St. Louis Association for Retarded Citizens.

Kart, C.S., Metress, E.S., & Metress, J.F. (1978). *Aging and health: Biologic and social perspectives.* Menlo Park, CA: Addison-Wesley.

Kaiser, H., Montague, J., Wold, D., Maune, S., & Pattison, D. (1981). Hearing of Down syndrome adults. *American Journal of Mental Deficiency, 85,* 467–472.

Keiter, J.B. (1979). Leisure activities and the AADD population. In P.J. Daniels (Ed.), *Gerontological aspects of developmental disabilities: The state of the art.* Omaha: University of Nebraska, Gerontology Program.

Krauss, M.W. (1986). *Long-term care issues in mental retardation.* Paper presented at the National Institute of Child Health and Human Development and Kennedy Foundation Conference, "Mental Retardation: Accomplishments and New Frontiers," Bethesda, MD.

Krauss, M.W., & Seltzer, M.M. (1984). *Aged-related differences in functional ability and residential status in mentally retarded adults.* Paper presented at the 108th Annual Conference of the American Association on Mental Deficiency, Minneapolis, MN.

Krauss, M.W., & Seltzer, M.M. (1986). Comparison of elderly and adult mentally retarded persons in community and institutional settings. *American Journal of Mental Deficiency, 91,* 237–243.

Krauss, M.W., Seltzer, M.M., Howard, A.M., Litchfield, L., & Post, D. (1986). *A national directory of programs serving elderly mentally retarded persons.* Waltham, MA: Florence Heller Graduate School, Brandeis University.

Kriger, S. (1975). On aging and mental retardation. In J.C. Hamilton & R.M. Segal (Eds.), *Proceedings: A consultation conference on the gerontological aspects of mental retardation* (pp. 20–32). Ann Arbor: University of Michigan.

Kriger, S. (1976). Geriatrics. In J. Wortis (Ed.), *Mental retardation and developmental disabilities: An annual review,* Vol. VIII. (pp. 156–167). New York: Brunner-Mazel.

Kultgen, P., Rinck, C., Calkins, C., & Intagliata, J. (1986). *Expanding the life chances and social support networks of elderly developmentally disabled persons*. University of Missouri-Kansas City: The UMKC Institute for Human Development.

Lakin, K.C. (1985). Service systems and settings for mentally retarded people. In K.C. Lakin, B. Hill, & R.H. Bruininks (Eds.), *An analysis of Medicaid's intermediate care facility for the mentally retarded (ICF/MR) program* (pp. 4-1 to 4-37). Minneapolis: University of Minnesota, Department of Educational Psychology.

Lakin, K.C., & Bruininks, R.H. (Eds.) (1985). *Strategies for achieving community integration of developmentally disabled citizens*. Baltimore: Paul H. Brookes.

Lakin, K.C., Hill, B.K., & Bruininks, R.H. (Eds.) (1985). *An analysis of Medicaid's intermediate care facility for the mentally retarded (ICF-MR) program*. Minneapolis: University of Minnesota, Department of Educational Psychology.

Lakin, K.C., Hill, B.K., Hauber, F.A., Bruininks, R.H., & Heal, L.W. (1983). New admissions and readmissions to a national sample of public residential facilities. *American Journal of Mental Deficiency, 88*, 13–20.

Lakin, K.C., Krantz, G.C., Bruininks, R.H., Clumpner, J.L., & Hill, B.K., (1982). One hundred years of data on populations of public residential facilities for mentally retarded people. *American Journal of Mental Deficiency, 87*, 1–8.

Landesman, S. (1986). Quality of life and personal life satisfaction: Definition and measurement issues. *Mental Retardation, 24*, 141–143.

Landesman, S. & Butterfield, E. (1987). Normalization and deinstitutionalization of mentally retarded individuals: Controversy and facts. *American Psychologist, 42*, 809–816.

Landesman-Dwyer, S. (1984). Residential environments and the social behavior of handicapped individuals. In M. Lewis (Ed.), *Beyond the dyad*. (pp. 299–322). New York: Plenum Press.

Landesman-Dwyer, S. (1985). Describing and evaluating residential environments. In R.H. Bruininks & K.C. Lakin (Eds.), *Living and learning in the least restrictive environment*. (pp. 185–196). Baltimore: Paul H. Brookes.

Landesman-Dwyer, S., Berkson, G., & Romer, D. (1979). Affiliation and friendship of mentally retarded residents in group homes. *American Journal of Mental Deficiency, 83*, 571–586.

Landesman-Dwyer, S., Sackett, G.P., & Kleinman, J.S. (1980). Relationship of size to resident and staff behavior in small community residences. *American Journal of Mental Deficiency, 85*, 6–17.

Larson, R. (1978). Thirty years of research on subjective well-being of older Americans. *Journal of Gerontology, 33*, 109–125.

Lott, I.T., & Lai, F. (1982). Dementia in Down's Syndrome: Observations from a neurology clinic. *Applied Research in Mental Retardation, 3*, 233–240.

Louis Harris and Associates (1979). *1979 Study of American attitudes towards pensions and retirement: A nationwide survey of employees, retirees, and business leaders*. New York: Johnson & Higgins.

Lowenthal, M.F., & Robinson, B. (1976). Social networks and isolation. In R.H. Binstock & E. Shanas (Eds.), *Handbook of aging and the social sciences*. New York: Van Nostrand Reinhold.

Lowy, L. (1985a). *Social work with the aging: The challenge and promise of later years*. Second edition. New York: Longman.

Lowy, L. (1985b). Multipurpose senior centers. In A. Monk (Ed.), *Handbook of gerontological services*. (pp. 322–340). New York: Van Nostrand Reinhold, Co.

Lubin, R.A., & Kiely, M. (1985). Epidemiology of aging in developmental disabilities. In M.P. Janicki & H.M. Wisniewski (Eds.), *Aging and developmental disabilities: Issues and approaches*. (pp. 95–114). Baltimore: Paul H. Brookes.

MacMillan, D.L. (1982) *Mental retardation in school and society*. Second edition. Boston: Little, Brown.

McConnell, S.R., Fleisher, D., Usher, C.E., & Kaplan, B.H. (1980). *Alternative work options for older workers: A feasibility study*. Los Angeles: Ethel Percy Andrus Gerontology Center.

Manfredini, D., & Smith, W. (in press). The concept and implementation of active treatment. In M.P. Janicki, M.W. Krauss, & M.M. Seltzer (Eds.), *Community residences for developmentally disabled persons: Here to stay*. Baltimore: Paul H. Brookes.

Mather, S. (1981). *Older developmentally disabled persons: The invisible senior citizen.* Madison, WI: Association for Retarded Citizens in Wisconsin.

Meiners, M.R. (1984). The state of the art in long-term care insurance. In P. Feinstein, M. Gornick, & J. Greenberg (Eds.). *Long-term care financing and delivery systems: Exploring some alternatives.* (pp. 15–34). Washington, D.C.: U.S. Department of Health and Human Services. (HCFA Publication No. 03174).

Meyers, C.E., Borthwick, S.A., & Eyman, R. (1985). Place of residence by age, ethnicity and level of retardation of the mentally retarded/developmentally disabled population of California. *American Journal of Mental Deficiency, 90,* 266–270.

Miniszek, N.A. (1983). Development of Alzeheimer disease in Down Syndrome individuals. *American Journal of Mental Deficiency, 87,* 377–385.

Mueller, B.J., & Porter, R. (1969). Placement of adult retardates from state institutions in community care facilities. *Community Mental Health Journal, 5,* 289–294.

National Association of Superintendents of Public Residential Facilities for the Mentally Retarded. (1984). *Directory of residential facilities for the mentally retarded.* Madison, WI: Author.

National Institute of Adult Day Care (1982). *Why adult day care?* Washington, D.C.: National Council on the Aging.

Neugarten, B.L. (Ed.) (1982). *Age or need? Public policies for older persons.* Beverly Hills: Sage Publications.

Neugarten, B.L., & Hagestad, G.O. (1976). Age and the life course. In R.H. Binstock & E. Shanas (Eds.), *Handbook of aging and the social sciences.* First edition. (pp. 35–55). New York: Van Nostrand Reinhold.

Neuman, F. (1981). *Ready, set; go—The institutionalized aging and aged developmentally disabled client: A new look at an old topic.* Paper presented at the 105th Annual Conference of the American Association on Mental Deficiency.

O'Connor, G., Justice, R.S., & Warren, N. (1970). The aged mentally retarded: Institution or community care? *American Journal of Mental Deficiency, 75,* 354–360.

Orbach, H.L. (1969). *Trends in early retirement.* Ann Arbor, MI: University of Michigan, Wayne State University Institute on Gerontology.

Pies, H.E. (1984). Life care communities for the aged—An overview. In P. Feinstein, M. Gornick, & J. Greenberg (Eds.). *Long-term care financing and delivery systems: Exploring some alternatives.* (pp. 41–52). Washington, D.C.: U.S. Department of Health and Human Services. (HCFA Publication No. 03174).

Puccio, P.S., Janicki, M.P., Otis, J.P., & Rettig, J. (1983). *Report of the committee on aging and developmental disabilities.* New York: New York State Office of Mental Retardation and Developmental Disabilities.

Reid, A.H. & Aungle, P.G. (1974). Dementia in aging mental defectives: A clinical psychiatric study. *Journal of Mental Deficiency Research, 18,* 15–23.

Richards, B.W. (1976). Health and longevity. In J. Wortis (Ed.), *Mental retardation and developmental disabilities: An annual review.* Vol. VIII. (pp. 168–187). New York: Brunner-Mazel.

Richards, B.W., & Siddiqui, A.Q. (1980). Age and mortality trends in residents of an institution for the mentally handicapped. *Journal of Mental Deficiency Research, 24,* 99–105.

Robins, E.G. (1981). Adult day care: Growing fast but still for the lucky few. *Generations, 5,* 22–23.

Robinson, P.K., Coberly, S., & Paul, C.E. (1985). Work and retirement. In R. Binstock & E. Shanas (Eds.), *Handbook of aging and the social sciences* Second edition. (pp. 503–527) New York: Van Nostrand Reinhold.

Romer, D., & Berkson, G. (1980a). Social ecology of supervised communal facilities for mentally disabled adults: II. Predictors of affiliation. *American Journal of Mental Deficiency, 85,* 229–242.

Romer, D., & Berkson, G. (1980b). Social ecology of supervised communal facilities for mentally disabled adults: III. Predictors of social choice. *American Journal of Mental Deficiency, 85,* 243–252.

Romer, D., & Berkson, G. (1981). Social ecology of supervised communal facilities for mentally disabled adults: IV: Characteristics of social behavior. *American Journal of Mental Deficiency, 86,* 28–38.

Rones, P.L. (1978). Older men—The choice between work and retirement. *Monthly Labor Review, 101,* 3–10.

Rotegard, L.L., & Bruininks, R.H. (1983). *Mentally retarded people in state-operated residential facilities: Years ending June 30, 1981 and June 30, 1982.* Minneapolis: University of Minnesota, Department of Educational Psychology.

Rowitz, L. (1980). *Survey of service use by the elderly retarded.* Paper presented at the Annual Meeting of the American Academy on Mental Retardation, San Francisco, California.

Scheerenberger, R.C. (1979). *Public residential services for the mentally retarded, 1979.* Madison, WI: National Association of Superintendents of Public Residential Facilities for the Mentally Retarded.

Scheerenberger, R.C. (1983). *Public residential services for the mentally retarded, 1982.* Madison, WI: National Association of Superintendents of Public Residential Facilities for the Mentally Retarded.

Scheerenberger, R.C. (1986). *Public residential services for the mentally retarded, 1985.* Madison, WI: National Association of Superintendents of Public Residential Facilities for the Mentally Retarded.

Schloen, K. (1984). An overview of home equity conversion. In P. Feinstein, M. Gornick, & J. Greenberg (Eds.), *Long-term care financing and delivery systems: Exploring some alternatives.* (pp. 81–82). Washington, D.C.: U.S. Department of Health and Human Services. (HCFA Publication No. 03174).

Schulz, J.H. (1980). *The economics of aging.* Second edition. Belmont, CA: Wadsworth.

Schulz, J.H. (1983). Private pensions, inflation, and employment. In H.S. Parnes (Ed.), *Issues in work and retirement.* (pp. 241–264). Kalamazoo: W.E. Upjohn Institute for Employment Research.

Segal, R. (1977). Trends in services for the aged mentally retarded. *Mental Retardation, 15,* 25–27.

Seltzer, G. (1985). Selected psychological processes and aging among older developmentally disabled persons. In M.P. Janicki & H.M. Wisniewski (Eds.), *Aging and developmental disabilities: Issues and approaches.* (pp. 211–227) Baltimore: Paul H. Brookes.

Seltzer, G.B., & Wells, A. (1986). *Generic day programs for seniors: An untapped resource?* Paper presented at the 110th Annual Conference of the American Association on Mental Deficiency, Denver, CO.

Seltzer, M.M. (1985). Informal supports for aging mentally retarded persons. *American Journal of Mental Deficiency, 90,* 259–265.

Seltzer, M.M. (1985). Research in social aspects of aging and developmental disabilities. In M.P. Janicki & H.M. Wisniewski (Eds.), *Aging and developmental disabilities: Issues and approaches.* (pp. 161–173). Baltimore: Paul H. Brookes.

Seltzer, M.M., & Seltzer, G.B. (1978). *Context for competence: A study of retarded adults living and working in the community.* Cambridge, MA: Education Projects, Inc.

Seltzer, M.M., Seltzer, G.B., & Sherwood, C.C. (1982). Comparison of community adjustment of older vs. younger mentally retarded adults. *American Journal of Mental Deficiency, 87,* 9–13.

Seltzer, M.M., Sherwood, C.C., & Litchfield, L. (1982). *A comparison of state regulations for community residences for mentally retarded persons, mentally ill persons, and elderly persons.* Paper presented at the 106th Annual Meeting of the American Association on Mental Deficiency, Boston, MA.

Shanas, E., & Sussman, M.B. (1981). The family in later life: Social structure and social policy. In R.W. Fogel, E. Hatfield, S.B. Kiesler, & E. Shanas (Eds.), *Aging: Stability and change in the family.* New York: Academic Press.

Sherman S.R., Frenkel, E.F., & Newman, E.S. (1984). Foster family care for older persons who are mentally retarded. *Mental Retardation, 22,* 302–308.

Sherwood, C.C., & Seltzer, M.M. (1981). *Analysis of board and care regulations.* Boston: Boston University of Social Work.

Sherwood, S., & Morris, J.N. (1983). The Pennsylvania domiciliary care experiment: I. Impact on quality of life. *American Journal of Public Health, 73,* 646–653.

Siegel, J.S. (1980). On the demography of aging. *Demography, 17,* 245–364.

Silverman, A.G., & Brahce, C.I. (1979). As parents grow older: An intervention model. *Journal of Gerontological Social Work, 2,* 77–85.

Silverstein, A.B., Herbs, D., Nasuta, R., & White, J.F. (1986). Effects of age on the adaptive behavior of institutionalized individuals with Down syndrome. *American Journal of Mental Deficiency, 90,* 659–662.

Snyder, B., & Woolner, S. (1974). When the retarded grow old. *Canada's Mental Health, 22,* 12–12.

Stone, R., & Newcomer, R. (1985). Health and social services policy and the disabled who have become old. In M.P. Janicki & H.M. Wisniewski (Eds.), *Aging and development disabilities: Issues and approaches.* (pp. 143–159) Baltimore: Paul H. Brookes.

Streib, G. (1983). The frail elderly: Research dilemmas and research opportunities. *The Gerontologist, 23,* 40–44.

Sutton, M.S. (1983). *Treatment issues of the elderly institutionalized developmentally disabled individual.* Paper presented at the Annual Convention of the American Psychological Association, Anaheim, CA.

Sweeney, D.P., & Wilson, T.Y. (1979). *Double jeopardy: The plight of aging and aged developmentally disabled persons in mid-America.* Ann Arbor: University of Michigan, Institute for the Study of Mental Retardation and Related Disabilities.

Talkington, L.W., & Chiovaro, S.J. (1969). An approach to programming for the aged mentally retarded. *Mental Retardation, 7*(1), 29–30.

Tarjan, G., Wright, S.W., Eyman, R.K., & Keeran, C.V. (1973). Natural history of mental retardation: Some aspects of epidemiology. *American Journal of Mental Deficiency, 77,* 369–379.

Tausig, M. (1985). Factors in family decision-making about placement for developmentally disabled individuals. *Journal of Mental Deficiency, 89,* 352–361.

Tobin, S., & Lieberman, M. (1976). *Last home for the aged: Critical implications of institutionalization.* San Francisco: Jossey-Bass.

U.S. Bureau of the Census. *Current Population Reports,* Series P-25, No. 930.

U.S. Senate Special Committee on Aging (1985–1986 Edition). *Aging America: Trends and projections.* Washington, D.C.: U.S. Department of Health and Human Services.

Von Behren, R. (1986). *Adult day care in America: Summary of a national survey.* Washington, D.C.: National Institute on Adult Day Care.

White, C.C., Hill, B.K., Lakin, K.C., & Bruininks, R.H. (1984). Day programs of adults with mental retardation in residential facilities. *Mental Retardation, 22,* 121–127.

Winklevoss, H.E., & Powell, A.U. (1984). *Continuing care retirement communities: An empirical, financial and legal analysis.* Homewood, IL: Richard D. Irwin, Inc.

Wolfensberger, W. (1985). An overview of social role valorization and some reflections on elderly mentally retarded persons. In M.P. Janicki & H.M. Wisniewski (Eds.), *Aging and developmentally disabilities: Issues and approaches.* (pp. 61–76). Baltimore: Paul H. Brookes.

Wood, J. (1979). Residential services for older developmentally disabled persons. In P.J. Daniels (Ed.), *Gerontological aspects of developmental disabilities: The state of the art.* Omaha: University of Nebraska, Gerontology Program.

Zetlin, A.G. (1986). Mentally retarded adults and their siblings. *American Journal of Mental Deficiency, 91,* 217–225.

Zigler, E., Balla, D. & Hodapp, R. (1984). On the definition and classification of mental retardation. *American Journal of Mental Deficiency, 89,* 215–230.

Index